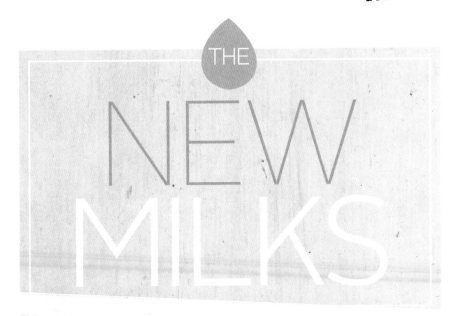

THE
NEW
MILKS

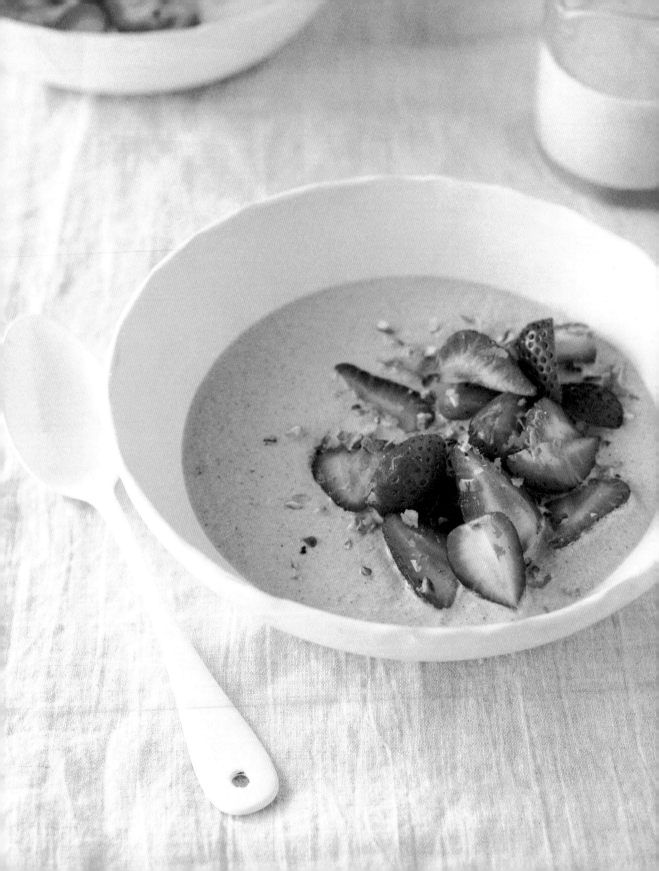

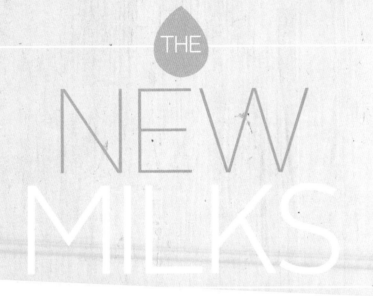

THE NEW MILKS

100-PLUS DAIRY-FREE RECIPES FOR MAKING AND COOKING WITH
SOY, NUT, SEED, GRAIN & COCONUT MILKS

DINA CHENEY

PHOTOGRAPHY BY SABRA KROCK

ATRIA PAPERBACK

NEW YORK   LONDON   TORONTO   SYDNEY   NEW DELHI

ATRIA PAPERBACK
An Imprint of Simon & Schuster, Inc.
1230 Avenue of the Americas
New York, NY 10020

First Atria Paperback edition May 2016

ATRIA PAPERBACK and colophon are trademarks of Simon & Schuster, Inc.

For information about special discounts for bulk purchases, please contact Simon & Schuster Special Sales at 1-866-506-1949 or business@simonandschuster.com.

The Simon & Schuster Speakers Bureau can bring authors to your live event. For more information or to book an event contact the Simon & Schuster Speakers Bureau at 1-866-248-3049 or visit our website at www.simonspeakers.com.

Interior design by Renata De Oliveira

Manufactured in the United States of America

10 9 8 7 6 5 4 3 2 1

Library of Congress Cataloging-in-Publication Data

Cheney, Dina.
The new milks : 100-plus dairy-free recipes for making and cooking with soy, nut, seed, grain, and coconut milks / Dina Cheney ; photography by Sabra Krock.
New York : Atria Paperback, [2016] | Includes index.
LCSH: Cooking (Nuts) | Soymilk. | Nut products. | Dairy substitutes. | Milk-free diet—Recipes. | LCGFT: Cookbooks.
LCC TX814 .C44 2016 | DDC 641.3/02—dc23

ISBN 978-1-5011-0394-0
ISBN 978-1-5011-0397-1 (ebook)

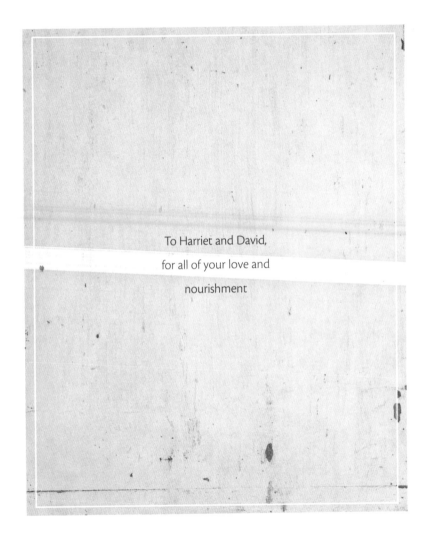

To Harriet and David,

for all of your love and

nourishment

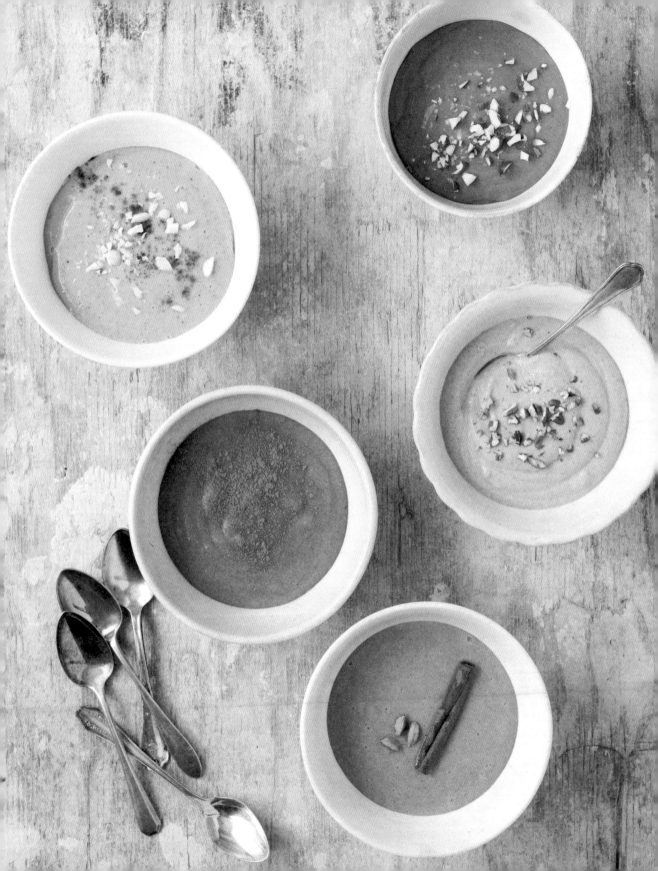

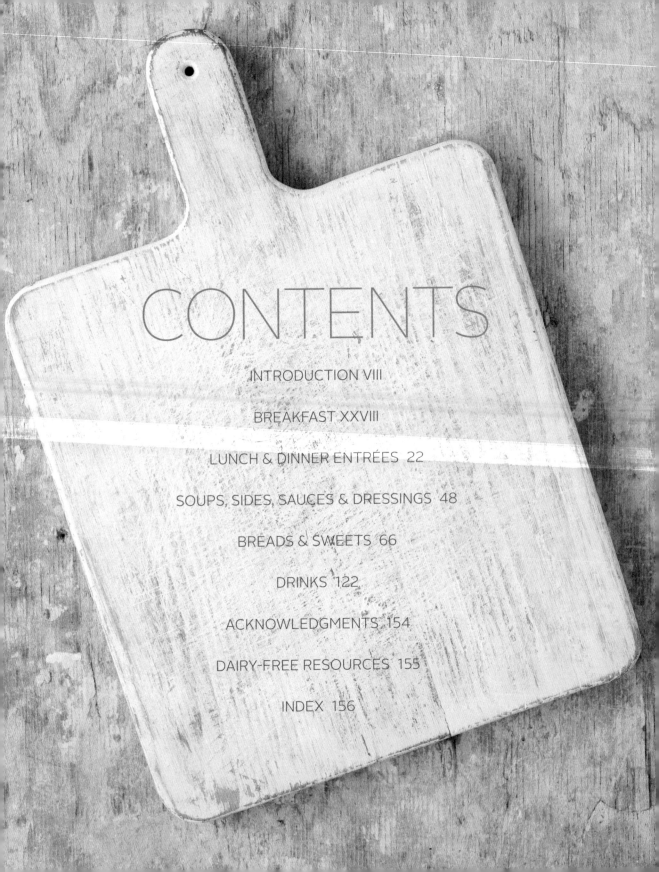

CONTENTS

INTRODUCTION

MEET THE NEW PLANT-BASED MILKS

A tall glass of cold milk: so simple and iconic. But gone are the days when milk always meant cow's milk, with its bright-white hue and aura of nurture and comfort. Today, the term could just as well connote a creamy beverage made from water plus nuts, seeds, legumes, grains, coconuts, or tubers. Although not a new invention, these plant-based milks (also known as alternative, vegan, or non-dairy milks) taste amazing, are as delicious as their base ingredients, and address many nutritional, philosophical, and culinary needs. Turns out there are at least fifty shades of white.

On the nutritional front, non-dairy milks are a boon for anyone who is lactose intolerant. This condition appears in people who lack the enzyme responsible for digesting lactose (the sugar naturally present in milk). When consuming dairy products—especially those that aren't fermented, namely milk—these people experience stomach discomfort and a variety of other symptoms.

Lactose intolerance is surprisingly common. The National Institutes of Health estimates that "approximately 65 percent of the human population has a reduced ability to digest lactose after infancy," with the condition especially prevalent among those of West African, Asian, Arab, Jewish, Greek, and Italian descent. According to the website for the U.S. Food and Drug Administration (www.fda.gov), "The National Institute of Diabetes and Digestive and Kidney Diseases estimates that 30 to 50 million Americans are lactose intolerant," including "up to 75% of all adult African Americans and Native Americans and 90% of Asian Americans."

Even if you aren't lactose intolerant, you may be one of the millions of people who follow a low-cholesterol, vegan, kosher, or Paleolithic diet. Or, perhaps you're allergic to dairy. If you fit into one or more of these categories, you'll find that non-dairy milks offer an exceptional alternative to dairy.

Philosophically, non-dairy milks represent a humane and ecologically sensitive choice. On many large dairy farms, female cows are separated from their young, constricted in small pens, and kept in a perpetual nursing state. When let out to graze, these same cows require ample land, and release significant amounts of methane gas into the atmosphere, which takes a toll on the environment.

Perhaps most important of all, plant-based milks are a cook's dream. They enrich our culinary arsenal, allowing us to tailor milks to specific recipes. We can use sweet and nutty hazelnut milk for porridges, thick coconut milk for ice creams, and creamy cashew milk for cream sauces.

Nearly every supermarket now stocks a selection of nut, seed, legume, grain, and coconut milks, and many coffee shops offer soy, almond, and coconut milks. However, if you want full control over the consistency and content of your milk, or wish to experiment with alternative flavors, you'll find that you can prepare your own batches with minimal effort.

Given all of these benefits, it's high time we broadened our definition of milk and explored the uncharted territory of plant-based alternatives!

THE NEW VERSUS THE MOO: A BRIEF NUTRITIONAL ANALYSIS

Although plant-based and cow milk are not identical nutritionally, they are comparable from a health perspective.

On the pro side, plant-based milks contain no cholesterol, lactose, or hormones. In general, they are loaded with phosphorus, potassium, folate, and magnesium just by merit of their nutritionally dense base ingredients. In addition, many varieties are high in calcium, vitamins, and minerals, thanks in large part to fortification. Pistachio nuts and pumpkin seeds are particularly high in protein, and nearly every seed milk is a good source of healthy omega-3 and omega-6 fatty acids. However, most packaged milks are strained and prepared with a low ratio of solids to water. As a result, they tend to be less nutrient-rich than their dairy counterparts. As Guy Crosby, science editor for America's Test Kitchen and adjunct associate professor at Harvard's T. H. Chan School of Public Health, puts it, "nut milks contain the contents of only a small number of nuts. So drinking an eight-ounce glass is equivalent to eating about four nuts."

The solution to this nutritional imbalance is to purchase fortified products, or prepare your own unstrained versions with higher ratios of solids to water.

To decide which milk alternatives are best for your particular needs, look over the chart on the next page, talk with your doctor, and consider any food allergies or health issues you have.

The chart on the next page compares the nutritional stats of some of the most popular and widely available packaged alternative milks, as well as their dairy counterparts. Keep in mind that the exact nutritional content of non-dairy milk varies from brand to brand. If you prepare your own unstrained milks and use a higher ratio of raw materials to water, you'll glean more nutrients.

NUTRITIONAL INFORMATION (PER EIGHT-OUNCE CUP)

	FIBER	PROTEIN	FAT	SATURATED FAT	SUGAR	CALORIES	CHOLESTEROL
Almond	0g	1g	2-3g	0g	0g	40	0mg
Cashew	0g	0g	3.5g	0g	0g	35	0mg
Coconut	1g	0g	4.5g	4g	0g	45	0mg
Flaxseed	0g	0g	2.5g	0g	0g	25	0mg
Hazelnut	1g	2g	3.5g	0g	0g	110	0mg
Hemp	1g	3g	5g	.5g	0g	70	0mg
Oat	2g	4g	2.5g	0g	19g	130	0mg
Quinoa	0g	2g	1g	0g	2g	70	0mg
Rice	0g	0-1g	2-2.5g	0g	0-1g	70	0mg
Soy	2g	7-10g	4.5g	.5g	2g	90	0 mg
Whole Milk	0g	8g	8g	5g	13g	146	24mg
Low-Fat Milk	0g	8g	5g	3g	12g	122	20mg
Skim Milk	0g	8g	0g	0g	12g	86	5mg

THE LAND OF MILKS AND HONEY: SHOPPING FOR PACKAGED MILKS

When I crave the freshest, purest, and most delicious milk, I make my own. However, I'm also a fan of packaged products, for convenience, smoothness (a boon when cooking), and long shelf life. While homemade milks last only three to four days in the fridge, packaged refrigerated milks can be stored for several weeks. Shelf-stable or aseptic milks keep for even longer—generally several months. These products are ideal for preparing the 113 breakfasts, lunches, dinners, desserts, breads, and drinks in this book.

Natural food chains, such as Whole Foods Market, tend to offer the most extensive selection of vegan milks. However, every major grocery store now stocks some. Look for perishable products in the refrigerated dairy section and aseptic boxes on the shelves.

What's in Packaged Milks?

Most packaged milks contain the ingredients listed below. Be sure to read the nutritional panel and ingredient list; if you avoid genetically modified organisms (GMOs), which are especially relevant when choosing a soy milk, purchase organic milk.

- **OILS AND THICKENERS** (xanthan, guar, gellan, and locust bean gums—which most studies have shown to be benign) make vegan milks thicker and creamier.

- **STABILIZERS AND EMULSIFIERS** (lecithin, carrageenan) prevent ingredients from separating and maintain consistency. While lecithin is derived from soy (and is an ingredient in most chocolate bars), carrageenan comes from seaweed. If you have a soy allergy or are concerned about carrageenan (some research has linked it to stomach upset), be on the lookout. As a result of the carrageenan controversy, Silk brand non-dairy milks no longer contain the ingredient.

- **SWEETENERS** (such as cane sugar) and flavors make milks taste good. After all, dairy milk contains lactose (natural milk sugar), while plant-based milks are, for the most part, very low in natural sugars. If you'd like to avoid these added sugars, make sure the word "unsweetened" appears on the package. (Most "original" versions include sweeteners.) I almost always opt for unsweetened, since such milks are healthier and more versatile. That said, flavored and sweetened products are delicious solo as a treat or incorporated into desserts and breakfast dishes, such as pancakes and bread pudding.

- **VITAMINS, MINERALS, PROTEIN, AND CALCIUM:** If you will be drinking non-dairy milk exclusively, purchase fortified milks or be sure to eat a well-balanced diet.

THE MILKY WAY: DIY PLANT-BASED MILKS AND CREAMS

Preparing your own vegan milks and creams is fun, easy, and low-tech. You'll be able to whip up a myriad of varieties and customize their tastes, textures, and nutritional properties. Countless methods abound, offering you lots of creative license, but the basic technique couldn't be simpler:

1. Soak solid ingredients (or not).

2. Rinse solid ingredients.

3. Cook, if necessary.

4. Combine solids with fresh water in a blender or food processor. Strain (or not).

Read on for details, including necessary equipment, plus tips and techniques.

The Equipment

For any non-dairy milk, you'll need the following:

- A large bowl

- A blender or food processor: High-speed blenders, such as the Breville Boss, are most effective at preparing plant-based milks, although food processors also work.

If you plan to strain (see "Blending and Straining" on page xiv), you'll also need:

- A nut milk bag, handheld fine strainer, unused panty hose, or a few layers of cheesecloth. Reusable nut milk bags, which will yield the most (and best-strained) milk, resemble a cross between cheesecloth and a pastry bag. Since they can be difficult to find in stores, you may need to order online, such as on www.amazon.com (they cost about ten dollars).

Differences between Coconut Milk, Coconut Cream, and Non-Dairy Creamer

COCONUT MILK comes in several forms. "Coconut milk beverage," akin to low-fat milk in terms of fat content, contains between 4.5 and 5 grams per cup. Look for it in refrigerated cartons or shelf-stable boxes. Meanwhile, light and full-fat "coconut milks" are intended for cooking, and come in cans (stocked in the Asian section) or in either refrigerated cartons or aseptic boxes (designated as "culinary coconut milk"). Full-fat coconut milk (canned or "culinary") contains 14 to 15 grams of fat per one third cup, compared to 5 grams for light.

Similar to whipped cream or whipped topping, "coconut cream" or "creamed coconut" contains about 3 grams of fat per tablespoon and makes an ideal base for vegan ice cream. Literally the fat that rises to the top of canned full-fat coconut milk, coconut cream is not synonymous with the sweetened "cream of coconut" used in cocktails. Unfortunately, it can be difficult to find. Order online (the brands Let's Do . . . Organic, Native Forest, and Aroy-D make it) or purchase at Trader Joe's or health food stores (call first to make sure stores carry it).

Otherwise, purchase a can of full-fat coconut milk whose contents do not slosh around when shaken (shake the can and listen to be sure). Then chill overnight. Open the can (do not shake first), and scoop the solid coconut cream off the surface. Or, make your own coconut cream from homemade coconut milk (see "Preparing Coconut Milk," page xvii). If you will be using canned coconut milk to prepare Whipped Coconut Cream (page 121), avoid brands that contain guar gum (at press time, Goya and Aroy-D canned coconut milk were free of the ingredient).

Several companies also make (sweetened) non-dairy creamers, typically based on coconuts, soybeans, almonds, or hazelnuts. Since these products—found in the refrigerated dairy section—are sweetened, I tend to avoid them.

For legume (i.e., soybean) and grain milks, you'll need:

- A saucepan
- (Optional, but helpful): A soy milk machine, such as the Soyajoy G4 Automatic Soy Milk Maker, which can also be used for preparing other vegan milks. At about one hundred dollars, the machine is cost-effective and will soon pay for itself.

For coconut milk made from whole coconuts, you'll need:

- A Phillips screwdriver
- A hammer, mallet, or rolling pin
- A dish towel
- A sharp paring knife
- (Optional, but helpful): A vegetable peeler

For preparing flour or meal out of leftover nut, seed, cooked legume, cooked grain, and coconut solids:

- **(Optional, but helpful): A food processor, such as the Breville Sous Chef**

The Raw Materials
Nuts and Seeds

- **Try hazelnuts, almonds, pistachios, pecans, walnuts, macadamia nuts, cashews, sunflower seeds, flaxseeds, pumpkin seeds, hemp seeds, and more.**

Start with any nuts out of their shells. You can use whole or sliced, blanched (i.e., no skins) or with skins (but avoid nut and seed flours). For seeds, opt for whole. Kayleen St. John, resident dietician at the Natural Gourmet Institute in New York City, and Dr. David Katz, director of Yale University's Yale-Griffin Prevention Research Center, both agree that whole nuts with skins supply more health benefits, as they're high in phytonutrients, flavonoids, fiber, and flavor. From a food science perspective, however, Guy Crosby argues that "the presence of skins makes it more difficult for the nuts to absorb water during soaking, slowing down the milk-making process." So, if you plan to use nuts with skins, allow for extra soaking and blending time.

When purchasing nuts and seeds, look for unsalted varieties, so you can control the flavor. I also prefer raw (unroasted), since they tend to be softer, enabling them to break down more easily (though you can use roasted nuts and seeds to create milks with deeper, more caramelized flavors). Visit the bulk section of your grocery store, and see what they have. Or go "shopping" in your pantry or freezer: I love to chill nuts, seeds, and whole grains in the freezer so they stay fresh longer.

Legumes

- **Try soybeans, mung beans, and more.**

Look for dried (raw) legumes in the bulk section of your grocery or health food store. If you're concerned about pesticides and GMOs, seek out organic or non-GMO soybeans (I order mine from www.nuts.com). Avoid flours.

Grains

- **Try quinoa, oats, wheat berries, millet, barley, farro, brown rice, and more.**

Use whatever grains you have on hand, but not leftover takeout rice, which can pose food safety issues. (Just make sure grains are cooked before using.) Although quinoa is technically a seed, treat it like a grain. If possible, purchase a prerinsed white variety, as it's lighter in hue and free of the hull's bitter coating. If it has not been prerinsed, make sure to rinse it. Do not use flour.

Coconut

- **Try whole or shredded coconut.**

Look for whole coconuts whose contents slosh around when you shake them (signifying the presence of coconut water). If you can't find whole coconuts, you can use unsweetened shredded or flaked coconut (look for directions on page xix), though the results are less than optimal. Do not use coconut flour.

Tubers

- **Try tiger nuts.**

Tiger nuts (*chufas*) are small tubers popular in West Africa and Spain, where they're used to make milk-like beverages called *kunnu* and *horchata de chufa*, respectively. They're available at some Whole Foods Markets and health food stores and at www.organicgemini.com. Soaking them before blending and straining will yield a naturally sweet, creamy white milk.

Combinations

Try mixing raw materials, such as coconut with almonds or different grains. Here are a few ideas:

- Coconut-almond, coconut-hazelnut, coconut-pistachio
- Hazelnut-almond
- Mung bean–soy (for a savory milk, excellent for stews, soups, and porridges)
- Brown rice–buckwheat (for malty pancakes), brown rice–millet

The Process

Soaking (Not Required for Coconuts and Small Seeds)

In most cases, you'll want to begin by soaking your solid ingredients. This is especially true for legumes, grains, and hard nuts, though you do not need to soak coconut or small seeds (such as flax or sesame). To soak, cover the raw ingredients with a couple of inches of water, and let sit at room temperature for at least eight hours. (Softer grains, such as oats, can soak for just a couple of hours.) Rinse and drain.

Why soak? According to Crosby, "when raw nuts are first soaked in water, the water is absorbed into the nuts, so subsequent grinding releases the oils (fat) as tiny droplets, which form a creamy emulsion. When the solid nut particles are strained off, the remaining liquid is similar to cow's milk, containing droplets of fat, proteins, sugars, and salts (minerals) dispersed in water. This step must be included to make a milk-like liquid." Some also feel that soaking removes or neutralizes the phytic acid present in most beans, grains and nuts, allowing the body to absorb more of their nutrients. (Coconut does not contain phytic acid, and does not need to be soaked.)

If you want to take soaking farther, try sprouting, which involves soaking the raw material in water, and rinsing repeatedly, until sprouts form or germination occurs. While St. John, Crosby, and Katz all agree that absorbable nutritional content tends to rise as a result of soaking and sprouting, there is little hard data on its effects. You can also purchase sprouted ingredients; look in the bulk section at Whole Foods Market and health food stores.

Cooking (Only Required for Legumes, including Soybeans, and Grains)

For milk that is easy to digest and tastes great, legumes must be soaked, rinsed, and cooked. I also highly recommend cooking grains for grain milks; doing so yields thicker, milder milks with rounded flavors. See the next page for details on cooking legumes and grains.

Blending and Straining

Although it's slightly pricier, I prefer a higher ratio of solid material to water (generally 1:2), for a more flavorful and creamier milk. Plus, I can always dilute later on, if necessary. To achieve a great result, blend on the "puree" setting until smooth (one or two minutes with a high-speed blender, and up to five minutes with a less powerful blender or food processor).

In general, the less water you use, the

thicker and more flavorful your milk will be, and the lower the yield. For strained milks, your yield should be similar to the amount of water you used. For unstrained milks, it should be about the same as the sum total of solids and water you used.

I generally recommend straining for milk, especially if you'll be using it in recipes, since doing so results in a more refined, milk-like liquid. (Do not strain for creams.) Note, though, that straining does remove many nutrients from the milk. If you're making a batch of milk to drink,

you may wish to leave it unstrained (and perhaps fortify it as well, as described on page xx).

To strain, position a clean nut milk bag over a large bowl or wide pitcher. Gather up the sides of the bag, and squeeze out the milk. You will most likely need to wring it out repeatedly (especially for legume milk). I've found that a nut milk bag will last for about ten uses, so make sure to keep more than one on hand. To clean the bag, turn it inside out and rinse very well. Keep your strained-out solids for use later on (see page xxi).

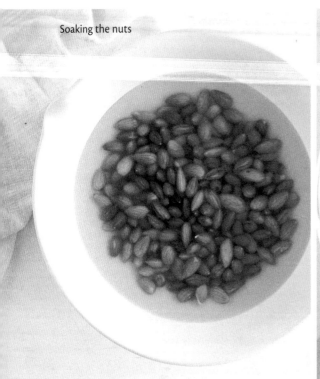

Soaking the nuts

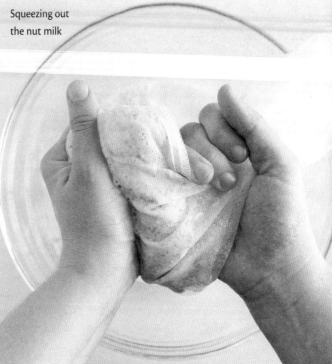

Squeezing out the nut milk

Achieving Thinner and Thicker Consistencies

- If you'd like thinner (more mildly flavored) milk, similar to 1% dairy or store-bought non-dairy products, use a lower ratio of raw material to water (such as 1:3 or 1:4), cold or room-temperature water, and raw ingredients lower in fat, starch, and fiber. For higher-fat seeds, such as flax, hemp, and sunflower (but not pumpkin), try a raw material to water ratio of 1:5 to 1:8. Otherwise, you'll yield milk more akin to a thick batter in consistency. Strain.

- If you'd like thicker (more flavorful) milk, similar to 2% dairy, use a higher ratio of raw material to water (such as 1:2), hot or boiling water, and ingredients higher in fat, starch, and fiber. (Be sure to hold down the blender lid when blending to avoid burns.) Do not strain. For even thicker milk, add the finished milk to a saucepan, bring to a simmer over medium-high heat, and then reduce the temperature and simmer for a few minutes on medium low (this also helps to prevent separation). You can also puree the finished milk in the blender with coconut oil, coconut butter, lecithin powder, or nut butter.

- If you'd like ultra-thick and flavorful creams, similar to whipped cream, use a 1:1 ratio (before soaking) of nuts to water. For oil-rich seeds, such as sunflower and hemp, opt for a ratio of 1:2 or 1:3. Remember to rinse and drain if you soaked, and to blend until smooth with fresh water (hot or boiling water will result in the thickest cream). Do not strain.

Special Considerations for Legume (Soybean), Grain, and Coconut Milks

Preparing Legume Milks

Allot enough time to prepare these milks, since the dried legumes must be soaked and cooked. For my two preferred methods, below, I start by soaking 1 cup of dried legumes, such as soybeans, in a few inches of water to cover overnight. Once fully soaked, the beans will have increased in volume to about 2¾ cups.

> **MACHINE, SUCH AS THE SOYAJOY G4 AUTOMATIC SOY MILK MAKER:** Rinse and drain the beans and add to the machine, along with the specified amount of water. Follow the machine's directions (the machine cooks the beans). The process should take about 25 minutes. For ultra-thick milk, do not strain. For smoother milk, strain (squeeze the nut milk bag several times). If you follow the machine's directions, you'll produce about 6 cups milk and 3 cups *okara* (soybean pulp).

> **MANUAL:** Rinse and drain the beans. Steam or boil until tender, about 1 hour. Add to a blender, along with 4 cups of water. Blend until smooth, about 2 minutes. If you strain (optional), you'll reap about 4 cups of creamy milk.

Preparing Grain Milks

I vastly prefer grain milks made with cooked grains. I've found that they develop a milder, more rounded flavor and a creamier texture. Raw grains will yield milk with a grassy, seedy, dirty, and bitter flavor, a chalky texture, and—sometimes—an off-putting aroma. Not very appetizing!

1. Rinse, soak, then rinse again.

2. Cook in fresh water, following the package

directions. Usually, you'll add the raw grains and water to a saucepan, and bring to a boil over medium-high heat. Cover and simmer over low heat until tender, between 20 and 60 minutes. All of the liquid should be absorbed by the grain (discard any cooking water that remains).

3. Blend cooked grains with the desired amount of fresh water. If you use a high ratio of grain to water and do not strain, the resulting milk can veer into porridge territory. Opt for a 1:2 or 1:3 ratio of cooked grain to water. Using boiling or hot water helps to release more starch and aroma molecules, for thicker and more flavorful milk.

4. Straining is optional. I never strain cooked oat milk, since the oats break down completely in the liquid.

Preparing Coconut Milk

Homemade coconut milk is incredibly nutty and sweet, especially if you use whole coconuts. Keep in mind that you cannot use coconut oil to prepare coconut milk (it's pure fat and, thus, lacks flavor).

IF USING WHOLE COCONUTS:

1. Choose two whole coconuts. Locate the end of each coconut that looks a bit like a face. With a Phillips screwdriver, poke holes in each fruit, one over each "eye."

   Invert the fruits, eyes side down, over a fine strainer placed over a bowl. Allow the coconut water to drain out. Pour the coconut water into a blender (you should yield about ⅔ cup per fruit).

2. Place the drained coconuts on a cutting board and cover with a large, clean kitchen towel. Thwack the fruit hard multiple times with a rolling pin, hammer, or mallet, until it cracks and breaks into several pieces. With a sharp paring knife, separate the white flesh from all of the brown matter. Then, use a vegetable peeler to remove any stubborn bits of brown skin that remain.

Rush Methods

IF YOU don't have time to soak your raw material, you can place solid ingredients in a high-speed blender, and blend for about 25 seconds (with nuts, don't let butter form). Add twice as much boiling water as solids. Blend for 1 minute. Let sit for 10 minutes, then blend for 1 more minute. Strain, if desired.

If you're really in a pinch, you can blend nut, seed, or coconut butter (not oil) with water, in a ratio of 1:8. Note, though, that this will yield much less flavorful milk.

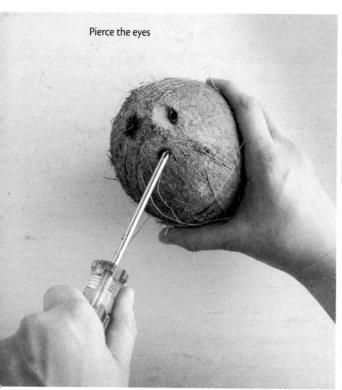
Pierce the eyes

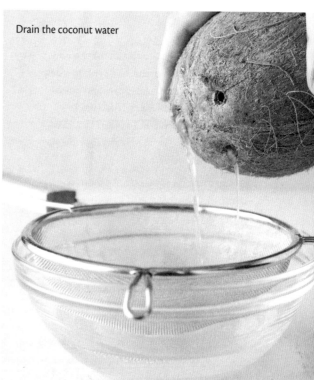
Drain the coconut water

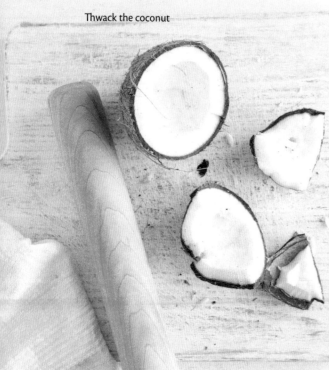
Thwack the coconut

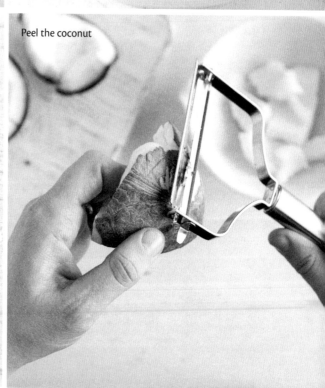
Peel the coconut

3. Break the white flesh into separate pieces (you should yield about 1½ cups per fruit), and add to the blender. To the 1⅓ cups of coconut water and 3 cups of flesh in the blender, add 2 cups of boiling or hot water. Hold down the blender lid, and blend until smooth, about 2 minutes. Strain. You should yield about 3½ cups milk from the two coconuts. Cover and chill.

If using shredded or flaked unsweetened coconut:

- Add 2 cups coconut to a blender, along with 4 cups of hot or boiling water. (Since coconut lacks phytic acid and breaks down easily, there's no need to soak.) Blend until smooth, about 1 minute. Strain. You should yield about 3½ cups milk. Cover, and chill.

With either method, after a couple of hours, you will notice that the milk begins to separate. Eventually, all of the fat (cream) will rise to the top. For homemade coconut cream, spoon off that entire top white layer. For full-fat coconut milk, stir the cream on top back into the rest of the liquid. For lower-fat coconut milk, remove some or all of the cream, add water to thin further, and stir.

Flavoring

If you plan to use your milk for several purposes, keep it unflavored for versatility. If you'd like to drink it solo or make a special version, try the additions listed below (I have included definitions for the more esoteric ingredients).

SWEETENERS

- Granulated sugar
- Agave nectar
- Pure maple syrup
- Honey
- POWDERED LUCUMA FRUIT: Powdered alternative sweetener derived from the lucuma fruit, grown in Peru, Chile, and Ecuador. With green skin and dry yellow flesh, the fruit resembles a cross between a mango and an acorn squash. The sweet off-white powder tastes like a cross between maple syrup and sweet potato.
- Whole pitted dates (need to be strained out)
- BROWN RICE, COCONUT, AND DATE SYRUPS: These brown-hued alternative sweeteners are similar in appearance and taste.

Preventing Separation

I'VE FOUND that many batches of milk do not separate. However, if they do, just shake before using.

Or, pour into a saucepan, bring to a simmer over medium-high heat, and then reduce the temperature and

simmer over medium low until the milk thickens slightly (watch carefully to make sure it doesn't boil over).

UNSTRAINED FLAVORINGS (DO NOT NEED TO BE STRAINED OUT AFTER BLENDING)

Since many of these ingredients have dominant flavors, use sparingly. Start with a small amount, such as ¼ teaspoon per serving, and increase from there. I rely on the Navitas Naturals brand for powdered lucuma, pomegranate, camu or camu camu, goji, maqui, and maca. Note that these ingredients are pricey, and a little goes a long way.

- Kosher salt
- Ground spices (cinnamon, nutmeg, cloves, ginger, pumpkin pie spice, cardamom, curry, saffron, turmeric)
- Unsweetened cocoa powder
- Espresso powder
- MATCHA: Powdered shade-grown Japanese green tea. Bright green hue and vegetal-grassy-floral flavor with subtle bitterness. Matcha is available in the tea section of most grocery stores (the Republic of Tea brand is distributed widely). For culinary purposes, you can use lower-grade, more economical products. Save very costly matcha for drinking solo. Look for powdered matcha (not in bags).
- ESSENCES (SUCH AS ORANGE AND ROSE FLOWER WATERS): Look for these bottled clear flavorings in international and ethnic markets, health food stores, gourmet grocers, and Whole Foods Markets.
- Pure extracts (vanilla, almond, hazelnut, etc., such as Nielsen-Massey brand)
- Tamarind paste, concentrate, or syrup
- SPIRULINA: Protein-rich blue-green algae dietary supplement available at health food stores.
- Powdered pomegranate
- POWDERED CAMU OR CAMU CAMU FRUIT: Red-orange powder with a tart berry taste, derived from the Amazonian berry.
- POWDERED GOJI: Made from the goji berry or wolfberry, native to China. The powder has a light orange hue and a sweet flavor tasting like a cross between raspberries and caramel popcorn.
- POWDERED MAQUI: Dark purple-brown tart-sweet powder made from a Patagonian fruit. Tastes like a cross between cranberries and pomegranate seeds.
- POWDERED MACA ROOT: Sweet, slightly bitter, nutty off-white powder from an Andean root. Tastes a bit like roasted parsnips.

- Vanilla bean seeds or paste (such as Nielsen-Massey brand)
- Syrups, such as pomegranate or sour cherry (also sweeteners)

STRAINED FLAVORINGS (NEED TO BE STRAINED OUT AFTER BLENDING)

- Flaked or shredded unsweetened coconut
- Grated citrus zest (colored zest only; no white pith)
- Fresh fruit, such as berries
- Pitted dates
- Fresh herbs, such as basil or mint

STEEPED FLAVORINGS

- Pesticide-free dried flowers, such as chamomile or hibiscus blossoms or rosebuds. Look for them in herbal and natural food stores and ethnic markets.
- Grated fresh ginger or turmeric root
- Tea leaves

Here are some guidelines for adding these ingredients:

- To make unsweetened drinking milk, add ⅛ teaspoon kosher salt per cup.
- To make sweetened milk, add ⅛ teaspoon kosher salt, 4 teaspoons sweetener, and ½ teaspoon vanilla per cup.
- Add unstrained flavorings to the finished milk. Blend (in the cleaned-out blender). Or, bring to a simmer to dissolve the ingredients.
- Add strained flavorings to the water and raw materials before blending. Blend, then strain.
- Add steeped flavorings to the finished milk, bring to a simmer, then strain.

The Leftovers

If You Strain, What Should You Do with the Solids?

One benefit of straining is the resulting wet, fiber-rich solids, which can be added to batters, smoothies, and oatmeal or baked and then ground into meal or flour.

How to Use Okara (from Soybeans)

Okara is the pulp left over from straining soy milk. Save the strained-out okara for sweet or savory dips and spreads, smoothies, stews, veggie burger patties, and quick bread batters. After all, the protein- and fiber-rich ingredient is appealingly creamy and adds bulk to dishes and baked goods. Or, follow the steps below to turn it into flour. Okara keeps well for up to two days in the fridge. One of these days, I intend to make a variation of Chinese red bean buns with sweetened okara!

How to Make and Use Meal or Flour

Store-bought meal and flour from ingredients such as coconut, hazelnut, and almond are very pricey. To make your own, pour the strained-out solids onto a parchment-lined rimmed baking sheet in one layer. Bake at 250 degrees F until dried out (but not brown), 2 to 3 hours. Grind into flour in a food processor, pulsing 60 to 80 times. In general, you should yield about ¾ cup from 1 cup of solids.

Use the meal or flour in baked goods, such as piecrusts, muffins, and cookie dough. Try substituting for about one quarter of the flour in recipes to add flavor and nutrients, such as protein, magnesium, or fiber. The meal keeps for up to four days in the fridge or a few months in the freezer.

A Rainbow of Plant-Based Milks in Your Kitchen

Generally, vegan and dairy milks can be used interchangeably in recipes. That said, non-dairy milks vary in flavor, hue, and thickness, due to different raw materials and preparation methods. When selecting milk for a recipe, taste it first to ensure that its flavor and color will mesh well with the other ingredients. For example, nutty, pale green pistachio milk wouldn't complement barbecued tofu. Also make sure that the milk has the right consistency. Usually this is only a problem when the milk is too thin; for example, rice milk would be too watery for a savory cream sauce.

FLAVOR AND USAGE CHART

The chart on pages xxiv–xxv summarizes the flavors, hues, and suggested uses for various plain unsweetened non-dairy milks. (I've left out milks I do not recommend preparing, including Brazil nut, chia seed, amaranth, peanut, and white sesame.) As with nutritional properties, qualities will vary depending on the preparation methods you use. I've attempted to be as comprehensive as possible with this table; however, it seems as if each day, we're introduced to a new ingredient. Try hosting your own plant-based milk tasting to determine your favorites!

WAYS TO ENJOY PLANT-BASED MILKS AND CREAMS

- Drink milks straight, either warm or chilled. Or add to cereal.
- Add milks to coffee or tea. Packaged full-fat coconut, cashew, and soy milks froth particularly well, as do homemade nut milks made with a 1:2 ratio of solids to water. I find that nut and grain milks taste best in coffee, since their flavors echo the nuttiness of coffee beans. Meanwhile, tea is delicious with soy, coconut, cashew, or almond milk.
- Dunk cookies in milks! My favorites, when I'm in a truly decadent mood, are sweetened cashew, hazelnut, or almond. When I'm feeling a bit more virtuous, I'll go with unsweetened nut, barley, tiger nut, or millet.
- Cook with milks, as used in the recipes in this book.
- Use creams as the base ingredient in sweet and savory dips, rich curries, puddings (as in the desserts on pages 108–118), milk shakes, and ice creams. Or, sweeten and dollop over fruit and sweets, instead of whipped cream, zabaglione, or pastry cream, as in Strawberries with Pistachio Cream (page 100). Creams can be savory (black bean), sweet (pistachio-almond), or more neutral and versatile (cashew).

TIPS AND TRICKS FOR COOKING WITH NON-DAIRY MILKS

- Since you can't buy vegan buttermilk, make your own—it's incredibly easy. Just stir 1 tablespoon of an acid (I tend to go for fresh lemon juice or cider vinegar) into 1 cup of vegan milk. Let sit for about 10 minutes at room temperature before using. Vegan buttermilk adds a complex, slightly tangy flavor and tenderness to baked goods (just make sure to use a bit of baking soda in the recipe). Feel free to substitute vegan buttermilk one-to-one for dairy buttermilk.

- To make your own vegan whipped topping, opt for Vanilla Almond Cream (page 119) or Whipped Coconut Cream (page 121). Try mixing different types of nuts, such as almonds and pistachios, the combination of which results in a slightly sweet, light green treat halfway between half-and-half and cream in consistency. For a dessert topping, you can substitute these vegan creams one-to-one for heavy cream or whipped topping.

- Since you can't buy vegan heavy cream or half-and-half, go for coconut milk (culinary or traditional canned, full-fat or light). When you don't want a coconut flavor, make a thick and mild alternative milk, such as cashew, macadamia, or soy (use a 1:1½ or 1:2 ratio of raw material to water).

- To make a vegan white or cream sauce, begin by melting vegan butter over medium heat in a skillet or saucepan. Once the butter is melted, whisk in flour until mixed well with the butter, about 30 seconds. Add a thick, mild non-dairy milk (such as cashew), and bring to a boil over medium-high heat. Reduce to a simmer, and cook, whisking, until thickened and smooth. Season. (For a Cajun-style roux, cook the butter-flour mixture until it becomes a bit darker in color.)

- To thicken puddings and smoothies, stir or puree the other ingredients with silken tofu; banana; vegan yogurt; lecithin; coconut oil; or coconut, nut, or seed butter. In addition, let dishes further set at room temperature or in the fridge.

- To prevent a skin from forming, as well as boilovers, watch simmering or boiling milk carefully, and do not let it boil for more than a minute or two. Also, use a saucepan that is relatively deep.

- Shake well before using, especially fortified vegan milks.

- Never freeze non-dairy milks.

THE RECIPES

HOW TO USE THESE RECIPES

This book includes 113 breakfast, lunch, dinner, dessert, bread, and drink recipes—some basics, such as Vegan "Creamed" Spinach with Garlic and Nutmeg (page 55) and Strawberry Shortcake with Fresh Lemon Zest (page 88), and others more creative, like Curried Cashew Pudding (page 112) and Avocado-Basil Smoothie (page 129). All are kosher and dairy-free, nearly 75 percent are vegan, nearly 60 percent are gluten-free, and many are Paleo. At the bottom of each recipe, when relevant, I include dietary tags and suggest alternate vegan milks to use.

Since many of you are exploring the world of alternative milks for health reasons, I have kept a large portion of these recipes nourishing and low on refined sweeteners and grains. That said, you *can* make recipes more decadent by simply adding a bit more sweetener and substituting all-purpose (white) flour for whole-grain. You can also swap white (granulated) sugar for coconut sugar or Sucanat.

In general, I recommend cooking with store-bought milks, since they're so convenient and, more importantly, contain stabilizers that prevent separation (much more attractive in finished dishes). That's why I developed all but a handful of these recipes with packaged milks (I clearly note when you need homemade milks).

FLAVOR & USAGE CHART

TYPE OF MILK	HUE	FLAVOR	SWEET/SAVORY	USES
Almond *	White to off-white	Mild; nutty	Sweeter	Especially puddings and coffee
Barley/Pearl Barley *	Off-white	Mild; nutty; beany; akin to soymilk	Sweeter	Especially warm sweet beverages and porridges
Cashew *	Off-white	Mild; nutty	Neutral	Especially good in creamy sauces, vegan cheeses, puddings
Farro	Off-white	Mild; very slight nuttiness and grassiness	Neutral	All, especially savory dishes
Flax	White to tan	Grassy	Neutral	All
Kamut *	Golden	Mild; rounded; beany; similar to rice milk; creamy	Sweeter	Oatmeal, porridge, drinking straight
Macadamia Nut *	White	Nutty; creamy	Sweeter	Especially good in desserts, cappuccino
Millet *	French vanilla	Mild; slightly nutty and beany; akin to soymilk	Sweeter	Drinking straight, oatmeal, desserts, smoothies
Oat (rolled, steel-cut, any other cut) *	Very white	Mild	Sweeter	Cereal, pudding, coffee
Pine Nut (Pignoli) *	White	Mild; nutty; slightly smoky; piney	Neutral	Especially good in Middle Eastern and Italian dishes, savory dips
Rice *	Very white	Mild; nutty (brown rice) Slightly floral (white rice)	Sweeter (Brown) Neutral (White)	Any, especially coffee and smoothies
Sorghum	Off-white	Mild; very slight grassy-sweet flavor	Neutral to sweet	Any, especially puddings, coffee, and drinking plain
Soy *	Off-white to pastry-cream	Mild; beany; most similar to cow's milk	Neutral	Most similar to dairy milk
Tigernut (Chufa) *	White	Nutty; milky	Sweet	Any, especially puddings, coffee, and drinking plain
Wheat berries	Off-white to beige	Mild	Neutral	Any, especially savory dishes

* Highly recommended alternative milk variety

TYPE OF MILK	HUE	FLAVOR	SWEET/SAVORY	USES
Black Bean	Light grey-purple-brown	Mild; beany	Neutral	Savory soups and stews, sweet and savory dips and spreads
Buckwheat	Light brown	Strong; nutty; beany; grassy	More savory	Savory crepes, savory oatmeal, bean stews, porridges
Coconut milk and cream *	White	Nutty; sweet coconut flavor	Sweeter	Asian curries, soups, and stews; pancakes, waffles, smoothies, milkshakes, ice cream
Hazelnut *	White	Mild; nutty	Sweeter	Desserts (especially chocolate and nut), smoothies, coffee
Hemp	Light brown	Grassy; bitter	Neutral	Chocolate- and strongly flavored sweets and baked goods (sweeten and flavor before use)
Mung Bean	Light olive green	Mild; pea soup–like	More savory	Savory soups and stews
Pecan *	Pale beige	Mild; nutty	Sweeter	Crepes and pancakes, cakes, soup or stew, brownies and other chocolate desserts
Pistachio *	Very pale green-tan	Mild pistachio flavor	Neutral	Gelato, pudding, cake, bread, smoothies
Pumpkin seed (pepita) *	Very pale green	Mild; slight smoky-pistachio flavor	Savory	Oatmeal, rice pudding, lasagna, mole, sauces, stews, soups, dips
Quinoa	Beige	Mild; chickpea-like	Neutral	Savory soups and stews, savory dips
Spelt/Freekeh	Spelt milk: beige to tan; freekeh milk: light green	Nutty, with a split pea-soup taste	Savory	Pea soup, savory stews
Sunflower	Beige to light tan	Appealing, subtle bitterness; nutty; tahini-like	Savory	Brownies, ice cream, yogurt, salad dressing, pumpkin soup, pancakes, dips, smoothies
Walnut *	White	Mild; walnut flavor	Neutral to sweeter	Pancakes, cakes, cream sauces, Greek and cinnamon-flavored desserts

That said, you can certainly try these recipes with homemade milks. To simulate store-bought, add a pinch more kosher salt and a bit more water, and shake the milk well or bring to a simmer before using.

Overall, know that with non-dairy milks—as opposed to cow's milk—there is a lot less consistency and standardization. Differences abound between store-bought and homemade, even between different brands of store-bought milk and different batches of homemade milk. I encourage you to keep tabs on which brands you prefer—for instance, I recently found that one of the almond milk products from a major grocery chain does not froth for coffee. For this reason, I wouldn't purchase it again.

THE NEW MILKS PANTRY

To prepare the recipes in this book, it's helpful to gather the following ingredients, which I've described or provided sourcing tips for, below. You might also want to stock up on some of the items in the Flavoring section on page xix and those in the Resources section (page 155). Whole Foods Markets and health food shops should carry most, if not all, of these items. If you don't have something on hand, you can always substitute with the easy-to-find, economical swaps I've listed.

- **KING ARTHUR WHITE WHOLE-WHEAT FLOUR:** This is 100 percent whole-wheat flour, but a milder, white-hued variety for a less wheaty taste and appearance. If you can't find it, opt for traditional whole-wheat flour or even all-purpose flour.

- **WHOLE-WHEAT PASTRY FLOUR:** This 100 percent whole-wheat flour is lower in gluten (wheat protein) than traditional whole-wheat flour, resulting in baked goods with a lighter texture and tender crumb. If you can't find it, use white pastry flour or traditional white or whole-wheat flour.

- **COCONUT SUGAR:** This brown sugar is derived from the sap of coconut blossoms. If you can't find it, opt for Sucanat or brown sugar (or white sugar). Make sure to use a small amount of baking soda when baking with coconut or other brown sugars, as these sweeteners contain some acid, which can affect the texture of baked goods.

- **SUCANAT:** Sucanat is the most coarse, unrefined form of brown sugar. As with coconut sugar, use a small amount of baking soda when baking. If you can't find Sucanat, opt for brown or coconut sugar (or white sugar).

- **AGAVE NECTAR:** Derived from the agave plant, this liquid sweetener is similar to honey, but vegan. If you can't find it, use honey, pure maple syrup, or sugar syrup (simmer equal parts sugar and water until the sugar dissolves). Feel free to use any type of agave nectar, whether raw, light, amber, or dark amber. As with maple syrup and honey, darker varieties have a bolder, more caramelized taste closer to that of molasses.

- **VEGAN BUTTER, SUCH AS EARTH BALANCE VEGAN BUTTERY STICKS:** I rely on this refrigerated product for sweet and savory dairy-free dishes. Use it just as you would a stick of butter. If you are not trying to avoid dairy butter, feel free to use it (just note that I developed my recipes with the vegan substitute).

- **GO VEGGIE! VEGAN PARMESAN CHEESE SUBSTITUTE:** This refrigerated vegan cheese (which comes in a small canister) is a respectable fill-in for Parmesan. If you are not trying to avoid dairy cheese, feel free to use traditional Parmesan or Parmigiano-Reggiano (just note that I developed my recipes with this particular product).

- **DRIED LEGUMES, NUTS, SEEDS, WHOLE COCONUTS, RAW GRAINS:** Visit the bulk section of your grocery or health food store, such as Whole Foods Market. You can also order dried organic (non-GMO) soybeans from many sources online, including www.nuts.com.

DIETARY DESIGNATION KEY

(V) Vegan

(VG) Vegetarian

(NF) Nut-Free

(GF) Gluten-Free

(P) Paleo-Friendly

BREAKFAST

ALMOND

MEXICAN FRITTATA WITH
CORN AND ZUCCHINI

"BUTTERMILK" ALMOND
WAFFLES WITH WARM
BERRY-AGAVE SAUCE

BAKED ALMOND AND
CINNAMON STEEL-CUT
OATMEAL WITH WARM
BERRY COMPOTE

VANILLA CHIA SEED
PUDDING WITH
COCONUT YOGURT

OAT

CHILLED DATE–
CINNAMON OATMEAL
WITH PECANS

OATMEAL PANCAKES
WITH TOASTED PECANS
AND RAISINS

TRIPLE APPLE OATMEAL
WITH MAPLE SYRUP

ORANGE CREPES

 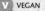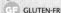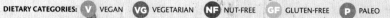

SOY

SCRAMBLED EGGS WITH
FRESH CHIVES

"CREAM CHEESE" WITH
PEPPER AND HERBS

CORNMEAL PANCAKES
WITH WARM
STRAWBERRY-RHUBARB
COMPOTE

RICE

HAZELNUT PANCAKES
WITH MOLASSES

HAZELNUT

CHERRY HAZELNUT
PANCAKES

CASHEW

FRENCH TOAST WITH
CINNAMON AND VANILLA

COCONUT

COCONUT FRENCH
TOAST WITH TROPICAL
FRUIT

DARK CHOCOLATE–
PECAN WHOLE-WHEAT
PANCAKES

MEXICAN FRITTATA WITH CORN AND ZUCCHINI

Mild almond milk gives this egg dish a smooth, custardy texture.
Opt for a high-quality salsa, or prepare your own. • **SERVES 6**

1 tablespoon plus 1 teaspoon olive oil, divided
1 cup finely chopped red onion (1 small)
1 cup finely chopped red bell pepper (about 1)
Scant ⅓ cup thinly sliced green onion, white parts only
2 teaspoons minced jalapeño
2 teaspoons minced garlic (1 large clove)
2½ cups thinly sliced (unpeeled) zucchini (about 1 medium-large)

1½ cups corn kernels (about 2 small ears)
½ teaspoon coarse kosher salt, divided
¼ teaspoon ancho or chipotle chile powder
8 large eggs
3 tablespoons plain unsweetened almond milk
¼ cup plus 1 tablespoon salsa
OPTIONAL FOR GARNISH: about ¼ cup finely chopped fresh cilantro leaves

PREHEAT the oven to 375 degrees F, and position a rack a few inches from the top. Brush the inside of a 10-inch nonstick skillet with half of the oil, and heat over medium high. When warm, add the red onion, bell pepper, green onion, jalapeño, and garlic, and sauté, stirring occasionally with a wooden spoon, until the bell pepper is tender, about 4 minutes.

STIR in the zucchini, and sauté until mostly tender, about 4 minutes. Add the remaining oil, plus the corn, half of the salt, and the chile powder. Sauté, stirring occasionally, until the zucchini is tender (but not overly soft), about another 2 minutes. With the spoon, evenly distribute the vegetables.

MEANWHILE, in a medium bowl, whisk the eggs with the almond milk and remaining ¼ teaspoon salt until smooth. Pour over the vegetables, and reduce the heat to medium. Continue cooking until the eggs set on the sides, 2 to 3 minutes. Spoon the salsa in about 15 dollops all over the top.

CAREFULLY transfer the pan to the oven, and bake until the egg mixture is cooked through, about 15 minutes. Let cool for about 10 minutes, garnish with cilantro if using, slice, and serve.

ALTERNATE MILK | CASHEW |

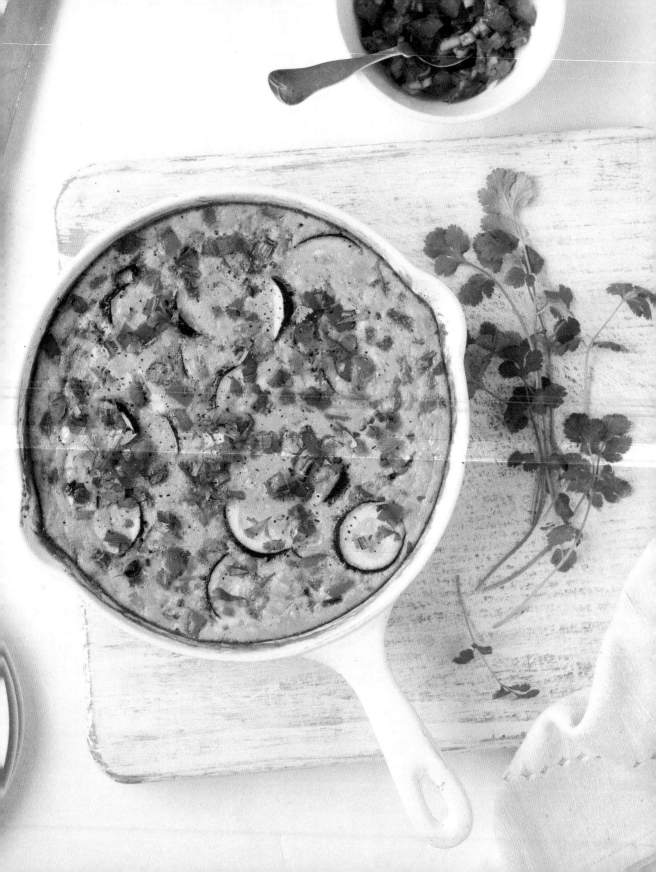

"BUTTERMILK" ALMOND WAFFLES WITH WARM BERRY-AGAVE SAUCE

These golden brown waffles are crisp and suffused with almond flavor. Feel free to garnish with lightly toasted slivered almonds. The batter is versatile and can also be used for pancakes. Before juicing, zest the lemons. • **SERVES 4 (MAKES 4 LARGE WAFFLES AND 1 CUP SAUCE)**

FOR THE WAFFLES

1¾ cups plain unsweetened almond milk

Scant 2 tablespoons fresh, strained lemon juice

2 tablespoons vegan butter, melted

1 teaspoon pure almond extract

1 teaspoon pure vanilla extract

1½ cups white whole-wheat flour

½ cup almond flour or meal

2 tablespoons coconut sugar

2½ teaspoons baking powder

½ teaspoon baking soda

½ teaspoon kosher salt

½ teaspoon freshly grated lemon zest

Cooking spray

FOR THE SAUCE

2 cups frozen mixed berries (strawberries, blueberries, raspberries)

½ cup agave nectar

1 teaspoon fresh, strained lemon juice

¼ teaspoon kosher salt

MAKE THE WAFFLES: In a large bowl, whisk together the milk and juice, and let sit for 5 minutes. Whisk in the melted butter and the almond and vanilla extracts.

IN A MEDIUM BOWL, whisk together the two flours, coconut sugar, baking powder, baking soda, salt, and zest. Pour the dry mix into the wet mix, and stir just until combined. Let sit for 15 minutes.

HEAT A WAFFLE IRON. When ready, spray with cooking spray, and prepare 4 waffles, according to your waffle maker's instructions. Spray the interior of the iron between waffles.

MEANWHILE, MAKE THE SAUCE: Add the sauce ingredients to a small to medium saucepan and bring to a boil over medium-high heat. Boil for 1 minute, and reduce the heat to low. Simmer until thickened and reduced to 1 cup, about 10 minutes. Serve the waffles with the sauce.

ALTERNATE MILK | COCONUT | HAZELNUT |

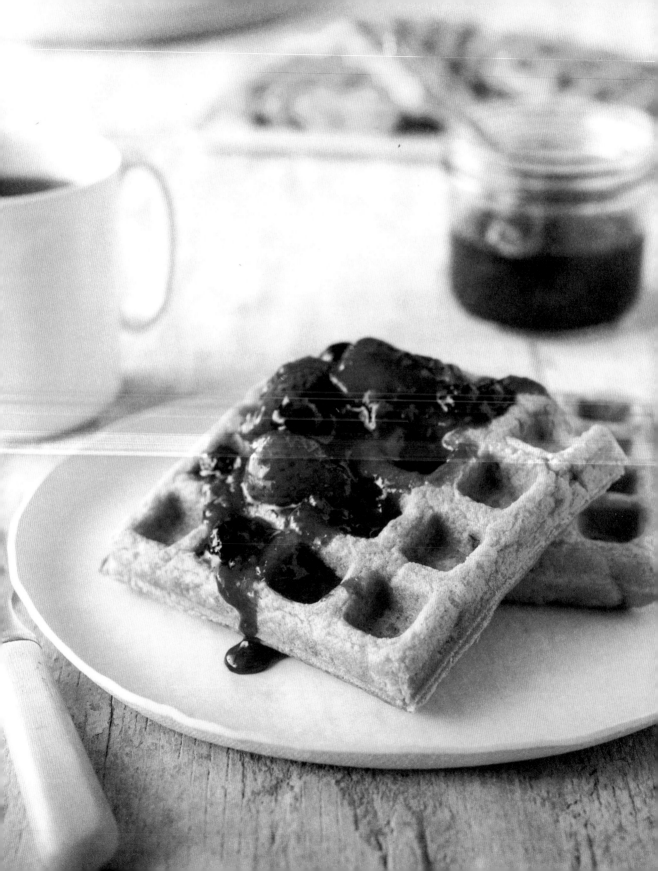

BAKED ALMOND AND CINNAMON STEEL-CUT OATMEAL WITH WARM BERRY COMPOTE

Crunchy toasted almonds and sweet berry compote make this breakfast special. If you're skipping the compote, stir in about a quarter cup of pure maple syrup. Don't skip the step of toasting the oats—it enhances their flavor. If reheating individual portions later, stir in more almond milk (about three tablespoons per serving). • **SERVES 6**

Cooking spray

1 tablespoon safflower or coconut oil

2 cups steel-cut oats

2½ cups unsweetened plain almond milk

⅓ cup creamy unsweetened almond butter

¾ cup plus 1 tablespoon pure maple syrup, divided

1 teaspoon ground cinnamon

1 teaspoon pure vanilla extract

1¼ teaspoons kosher salt, divided

3½ cups boiling water

2 cups berries

¼ teaspoon pure almond extract

¼ cup blanched slivered almonds, lightly toasted

PREHEAT the oven to 375 degrees F. Grease the inside of a roughly 13 x 9-inch baking dish with cooking spray. Brush the inside of a 10-inch non-stick skillet with the oil, and heat over medium. When warm, add the oats and cook, stirring occasionally, until aromatic and slightly golden brown, about 4 minutes. Set aside off the heat.

MEANWHILE, in a large bowl, whisk together the almond milk, almond butter, ¼ cup plus 1 tablespoon of the maple syrup, the cinnamon, the vanilla, 1 teaspoon of the salt, and the boiling water. Stir in the toasted oats, and mix well. Pour into the greased baking dish and carefully transfer to the center rack of the oven. Bake until the oats

are tender, about 1 hour. Remove the baking dish from the oven and stir the mixture well.

MEANWHILE, add the berries, the remaining ½ cup maple syrup, and the remaining ¼ teaspoon salt to a medium saucepan; stir; and bring to a boil over medium-high heat. Boil until thickened, about 10 minutes (watch the pan carefully, and remove it from the heat immediately once the mixture is reduced to 1 cup). Stir in the almond extract.

LADLE the warm baked oatmeal into 6 bowls. Divide the compote and toasted nuts among them. Serve immediately.

Gluten-free if using gluten-free oats

ALTERNATE MILK | COCONUT |

VANILLA CHIA SEED PUDDING WITH COCONUT YOGURT

Chia seed pudding has become popular in health-oriented restaurants—for good reason. It's incredibly easy to make, and delicious. Basically, stir together a handful of ingredients, and let the chia seeds naturally thicken the mixture into a nourishing, creamy pudding. Top with fresh fruit and nuts. ● **MAKES ABOUT 2¾ CUPS (3-4 SERVINGS)**

2 cups plain unsweetened almond milk

¼ cup agave nectar

¼ cup chia seeds

2 teaspoons pure vanilla extract

⅛ teaspoon salt

½ cup unsweetened plain coconut milk yogurt

ADD all of the ingredients except the yogurt to a quart-size jar. Place the lid on, and shake well. Chill overnight (the pudding will thicken a bit). Stir in the yogurt, and serve.

ALTERNATE MILK | COCONUT | CASHEW |

CHILLED DATE-CINNAMON OATMEAL WITH PECANS

It sounds counterintuitive, but chilled (rather than hot) oatmeal—similar to muesli—is smooth, rich, creamy, and flavorful. For the ultimate texture, don't skip the step of soaking the raw oats overnight (it enables them to soften). I love to make a large batch and keep it in the fridge for up to five days. ● **MAKES 3½ CUPS (ABOUT 4 SERVINGS)**

2 cups rolled oats
1 cup plain unsweetened oat milk
10 pitted dates
½ cup whole pecans
1 tablespoon pure maple syrup

2 teaspoons pure vanilla extract
1 teaspoon ground cinnamon
½ teaspoon kosher salt
Optional for garnish: fresh berries

POUR the oats into a medium bowl, and cover with 4 cups lukewarm water. Cover and let soak overnight. Rinse and drain.

ADD the oats to a high-speed blender, along with the oat milk, dates, pecans, maple syrup, vanilla, cinnamon, and salt. Puree until smooth, about 40 seconds. Ladle into 4 small bowls, and top with berries.

Gluten-free if using gluten-free oats

ALTERNATE MILK | COCONUT | ALMOND |

OATMEAL PANCAKES WITH TOASTED PECANS AND RAISINS

Inspired by a bowl of oatmeal with nuts, raisins, and cinnamon, these pancakes can be doubled for brunch get-togethers. To convert to vegan, use an egg substitute or one tablespoon of ground flaxseeds mixed with water.

● SERVES 5 TO 6 (MAKES ABOUT 20 SMALL PANCAKES)

1¾ cups plain unsweetened oat milk
Scant 2 tablespoons orange juice
3 tablespoons safflower oil, divided
1 large egg
2 teaspoons pure vanilla extract
1½ cups white whole-wheat flour
1 cup plain quick oats
2 tablespoons Sucanat or brown sugar

1½ teaspoons baking powder
1 teaspoon ground cinnamon
½ teaspoon baking soda
½ teaspoon kosher salt
½ cup raisins, ideally a mix of purple and golden
½ cup pecans, lightly toasted and finely chopped

STIR together the milk and juice in a large bowl, and let sit for 10 minutes. Then, stir in 2 tablespoons of the oil, the egg, and the vanilla. Meanwhile, add the next seven ingredients to a medium bowl, and whisk well. Pour the dry mixture into the wet mixture, and stir just until combined. Let the batter sit for about 15 minutes.

BRUSH the inside of a 10-inch nonstick skillet with the remaining tablespoon of oil, and heat over medium. When warm, add four scant

¼-cupfuls of batter, spacing them apart; sprinkle about 1 teaspoon each of the raisins and pecans onto each pancake.

COOK until they puff up around the edges and a few bubbles form, about 3 minutes. With a nonstick spatula, carefully flip and cook until the second side is fully cooked through, about another 3 minutes. Repeat with the remaining batter, nuts, and raisins (later batches will likely cook in slightly less time).

ALTERNATE MILK | COCONUT | CASHEW |

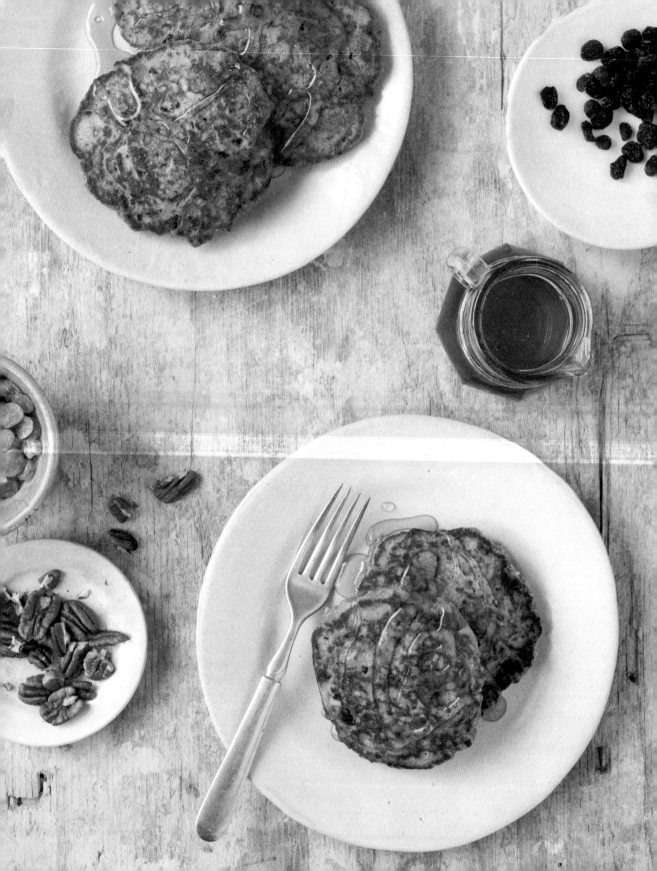

TRIPLE APPLE OATMEAL WITH MAPLE SYRUP

For another hit of apple, garnish with apple chips. • **SERVES 4**

2 cups apple cider
2 cups plain unsweetened oat milk
½ teaspoon kosher salt
½ teaspoon plus ⅛ teaspoon ground
 cinnamon, divided

2 cups rolled oats
1 cup shredded peeled apple, such as Fuji
 (about 2 apples)
¼ cup pure maple syrup
1 cup small dice unpeeled apple, such as Fuji

ADD the cider, oat milk, salt, and ½ teaspoon of the cinnamon to a medium saucepan; stir; and bring to a boil over medium-high heat. Stir in the oats and shredded apple, and cook uncovered over medium heat until thickened, about 2 minutes, stirring frequently.

STIR in the maple syrup. Cover and let sit off of the heat until thickened and the oats and apple are cooked through, about 5 minutes.

STIR again. Ladle into 4 small bowls, and sprinkle with the diced apple and remaining ⅛ teaspoon cinnamon.

Gluten-free if using gluten-free oats

ALTERNATE MILK | **ALMOND** | **CASHEW** |

ORANGE CREPES

Serve slathered with orange marmalade or strawberry preserves or drizzled with maple syrup or dairy-free dark chocolate sauce (try one teaspoon per crepe). Keep flat, roll up, or fold into quadrants. Consider preheating the oven to 300 degrees F to keep already-cooked crepes warm. ● **SERVES 4 (MAKES 9 CREPES)**

1¼ cups plain unsweetened oat milk
½ cup white whole-wheat flour
½ cup all-purpose flour
2 large eggs
2 tablespoons coconut sugar or brown sugar
1 teaspoon pure vanilla extract

½ teaspoon orange flower water or pure orange extract
¼ teaspoon kosher salt
About 1 tablespoon plus 2 teaspoons safflower oil for cooking, divided

ADD the first eight ingredients to a blender, and pulse until well combined, about 15 times. Chill for 1 hour.

WHEN ready to cook, heat a small nonstick sauté or crepe pan over medium heat, and brush with 1 teaspoon of the oil. When hot, pour in ¼ cup of the batter, and rotate the pan until the mixture spreads out. After about 5 seconds, use a small offset spatula to loosen the outside edges of the crepe from the pan. Once small bubbles have formed in the center (after 30 to 60 seconds of cooking), use a thin nonstick spatula to carefully

flip. Cook the other side for another 10 seconds, and flip onto a cutting board. Cover the crepe with a piece of parchment paper or a paper towel. (The first couple of crepes are never the prettiest.)

BRUSH the pan with another ½ teaspoon of the oil and add another ¼ cup of batter. Repeat the cooking process as described above, remembering to place a piece of parchment or a paper towel between each crepe on the cutting board. Serve warm.

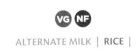

ALTERNATE MILK | RICE |

SCRAMBLED EGGS WITH FRESH CHIVES

Adding a bit of soy milk to eggs makes them fluffier, while chives provide fresh flavor and verdant color. Opt for a wooden spoon or silicone spatula to avoid scratching your nonstick pan. • **SERVES 4**

2 tablespoons vegan butter
8 large eggs
¼ cup minced fresh chives

3 tablespoons plain unsweetened soy milk, well shaken
¼ teaspoon kosher salt
5 grinds black pepper

MELT the butter in a 10-inch nonstick skillet over medium heat. Meanwhile, in a medium-large bowl, whisk together the remaining ingredients until well blended.

ONCE the butter has melted, reduce the heat to medium low, and add the egg mixture.

COOK, occasionally scraping the eggs from the perimeter of the pan to the center and letting the liquid-y eggs take their place. (Do not break up the eggs with the spatula; keep them in large fluffy curds.)

REMOVE the pan from the heat when the eggs are about 90 percent cooked, as they will continue to cook.

ALTERNATE MILK | CASHEW | RICE |

"CREAM CHEESE" WITH PEPPER AND HERBS

Slather this buttery spread onto toasted bagels, rye or pumpernickel bread, or crackers. Top with thinly sliced cucumbers or smoked salmon. Feel free to vary the recipe by, say, adding shredded fresh carrots, minced red onion or shallot, or thinly sliced green onion.

● **MAKES A GENEROUS ¾ CUP**

¾ cup plain silken tofu (about half of a 14-ounce package), drained

¼ cup fresh herbs, such as chives, mint, basil, flat-leaf parsley, or cilantro, chopped finely

2 tablespoons plain unsweetened soy milk

1 teaspoon fresh, strained lemon juice

¼ teaspoon kosher salt

4 grinds black pepper

ADD all of the ingredients to a mini food processor, and puree until smooth, about 40 seconds. (Make sure that all of the herbs have been chopped fine.)

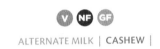

ALTERNATE MILK | CASHEW |

CORNMEAL PANCAKES WITH WARM STRAWBERRY-RHUBARB COMPOTE

Here, a chunky compote of gorgeous, in-season strawberries and rhubarb tops light and fluffy cornmeal pancakes. • **SERVES 6 (MAKES 24 PANCAKES AND 3½ CUPS COMPOTE)**

FOR THE PANCAKES

3 large eggs, separated

1½ cups unsweetened plain soy milk

2 tablespoons safflower oil, plus extra for cooking pancakes, divided

1 tablespoon vanilla extract

1 cup fine cornmeal or corn flour

1 cup all-purpose flour

3 tablespoons granulated sugar

2 teaspoons baking powder

¾ teaspoon salt

IN a standing mixer, beat the egg whites over medium-high speed until soft peaks form, about 7 minutes. In a large bowl, whisk together egg yolks, milk, 2 tablespoons of the oil, and the vanilla. In a medium bowl, whisk together the cornmeal, flour, sugar, baking powder, and salt. Pour this dry mixture into the egg yolk mixture, and stir just until combined. With a rubber spatula, fold in the whipped egg whites in thirds, just until combined.

BRUSH the inside of a 10-inch nonstick skillet with some safflower oil (about 1 tablespoon), and heat over medium high. When hot, add four ¼-cupfuls of batter. Cook until light golden on the first side, about two minutes. Flip and cook the other side until also golden brown, about another two minutes. Continue with the remaining pancakes, brushing with a teaspoon of oil between batches.

FOR THE COMPOTE

4 cups sliced fresh rhubarb

3 cups sliced fresh strawberries

½ cup maple syrup

1 teaspoon salt

ADD all of the ingredients to a medium saucepot, and bring to a boil over medium-high heat. Cook until the rhubarb is tender, about 15 minutes.

ALTERNATE MILK | ALMOND | CASHEW |

HAZELNUT PANCAKES WITH MOLASSES

Molasses lends these tender, moist pancakes a rich, toasty flavor.

● **SERVES 4 (MAKES 11 PANCAKES)**

1¾ cups plain unsweetened rice milk

2 large eggs

4 tablespoons vegan butter, melted

1 teaspoon molasses

½ teaspoon hazelnut extract

1 cup white whole-wheat flour

½ cup hazelnut or almond meal or flour

3 tablespoons coconut sugar or brown sugar

1 teaspoon baking powder

½ teaspoon kosher salt

1 tablespoon plus 1 teaspoon safflower oil,
   divided

IN a large bowl, whisk together the rice milk, eggs, vegan butter, molasses, and hazelnut extract. In a medium bowl, whisk together the whole-wheat flour, hazelnut flour, coconut sugar, baking powder, and salt.

BRUSH the inside of a 10-inch nonstick skillet with half of the oil, and heat over medium. When hot, add four ¼-cupfuls of batter to the pan. Cook until the edges puff up and you can see a few bubbles atop the pancakes, about 4 minutes.

FLIP with a nonstick spatula, and cook until the other side is golden brown and the centers are cooked through, about another 3 minutes. Repeat with the remaining oil and two other batches, keeping in mind that future batches will likely take 5 to 6 minutes total.

SERVE alone or with maple syrup, more molasses, or a mixture of softened vegan butter, fresh orange zest, and maple syrup.

ALTERNATE MILK | HAZELNUT | ALMOND |

CHERRY HAZELNUT PANCAKES

If you use unsweetened milk, add about one and a half teaspoons more Sucanat. Feel free to garnish with chopped toasted hazelnuts and to serve with maple syrup (though you shouldn't need it). ● **SERVES 4 (MAKES ABOUT 15 SMALL PANCAKES)**

2 cups spelt or whole-wheat flour
2 tablespoons Sucanat or brown sugar
1 tablespoon baking powder
Scant ¾ teaspoon kosher salt
1¾ cups plain hazelnut milk (sweetened)

2 tablespoons coconut butter, melted
1 teaspoon pure vanilla extract
1 teaspoon pure hazelnut extract
1 tablespoon (or more) safflower oil
2 cups fresh cherries, pitted and halved

IN a medium-large bowl, whisk together the spelt flour, Sucanat, baking powder, and salt. In a small to medium bowl, whisk together hazelnut milk, coconut butter, vanilla extract, and hazelnut extract. Add the wet ingredients to the dry, and mix just until combined. Let sit for 10 to 15 minutes.

BRUSH the inside of a 10-inch nonstick skillet with the oil, and heat over medium. When warm, add four scant ¼-cupfuls of batter, spacing them

apart; place about three cherry halves on each pancake.

COOK until the pancakes puff up around the edges and a few bubbles form, about 3 minutes. With a nonstick spatula, carefully flip and cook until the second side is fully cooked through, about another 3 minutes. Repeat with the remaining batter and cherries (the second and later pancake batches will likely cook in slightly less time).

ALTERNATE MILK | **PLAIN SWEETENED RICE** |

FRENCH TOAST WITH CINNAMON AND VANILLA

Serve with fresh berries and extra maple syrup. If you like, preheat the oven to 300 degrees F and keep cooked French toast warm while you finish preparing the dish. A serrated knife makes quick work of slicing the challah bread. • **SERVES 4 (MAKES 12 SLICES)**

1½ cups plain unsweetened cashew milk

3 large eggs

3 tablespoons pure maple syrup, plus extra for serving

1 teaspoon pure vanilla extract

1 teaspoon ground cinnamon

¼ teaspoon kosher salt

1-pound loaf challah or brioche, cut on the diagonal into twelve ½-inch-thick slices

About ¼ cup safflower oil, divided

IN a large bowl, whisk together the cashew milk, eggs, maple syrup, vanilla, cinnamon, and salt. One at a time, dip each slice of bread in the mixture, turning over to coat both sides. Shake off excess custard, and transfer the coated bread slices to a baking sheet or cutting board.

BRUSH the inside of a 10-inch skillet (nonstick or regular) with about 1 tablespoon of the oil, and heat over medium high. When hot, add 3 pieces of the coated French toast and cook until golden brown and slightly crispy on both sides, about 4 minutes. Transfer to a plate, and repeat with the remaining French toast, adding another tablespoon of oil with each new batch.

SERVE with fruit and maple syrup.

For a gluten-free version, prepare with gluten-free bread.

ALTERNATE MILK | COCONUT | ALMOND |

COCONUT FRENCH TOAST WITH TROPICAL FRUIT

Here, coconut cream and a tropical fruit salad enhance a rum-infused French toast.

● SERVES 4 (MAKES 12 SLICES)

2 cups diced pineapple

1 cup diced kiwi

1 cup diced mango or papaya

2 cups unsweetened coconut milk beverage

3 large eggs

3 tablespoons pure maple syrup, plus extra for serving

2 tablespoons white rum

1 teaspoon pure coconut extract or vanilla extract

½ teaspoon kosher salt

1-pound loaf challah or brioche, cut diagonally into twelve ½-inch-thick slices

About 2 tablespoons plus 1 teaspoon coconut oil, divided

¼ cup coconut cream

2 tablespoons unsweetened coconut flakes

IN a medium bowl, stir together the pineapple, kiwi, and mango.

IN a large bowl, whisk together the coconut milk, eggs, the 3 tablespoons of maple syrup, the rum, the coconut extract, and the salt. One at a time, dip each slice of bread in the mixture, turning over to coat both sides. Shake off excess custard, and transfer the coated bread slices to a baking sheet or cutting board.

BRUSH the inside of a 10-inch skillet (nonstick or regular) with about 2 teaspoons of the oil, and

heat over medium high. When hot, add 3 pieces of the coated French toast and cook until golden brown and slightly crispy on both sides, about 4 minutes. Transfer to a plate, and repeat with the remaining French toast, adding another table-spoon of oil with each new batch.

ONTO each of 4 plates, place 3 pieces of French toast. Top with 1 tablespoon of the coconut cream and one quarter of the fruit salad. Sprinkle with ½ tablespoon of the coconut flakes. Serve with extra maple syrup, if desired.

For a gluten-free version, prepare with gluten-free bread.

ALTERNATE MILK | CANNED FULL-FAT OR CULINARY COCONUT MILK |

DARK CHOCOLATE–PECAN WHOLE-WHEAT PANCAKES

Try dousing these pancakes with maple syrup or melted dark chocolate.

● **SERVES 4**

2 cups white whole-wheat or whole-wheat flour

2 tablespoons granulated sugar

2 teaspoons baking powder

¾ teaspoon salt

1¾ cups plain unsweetened coconut milk, canned or refrigerated beverage

2 large eggs

2 tablespoons safflower oil, plus extra for cooking pancakes, divided

1 teaspoon vanilla extract

About 3 ounces dark chocolate (preferably around 60 percent cacao content), chopped

½ cup finely chopped toasted pecans

About 12 ounces fresh blueberries and raspberries, for serving

IN a medium bowl, whisk together flour, sugar, baking powder, and salt. In a large bowl, whisk together milk, eggs, 2 teaspoons of the safflower oil, and vanilla. Pour the dry mixture into the wet mixture, and stir just until combined. Add the chocolate and pecans, and stir just until combined.

BRUSH the inside of a 10-inch nonstick skillet with 1 tablespoon of the oil, and heat over medium. When warm, add three or four quarter-cup dollops of batter, and cook until the first side is golden brown, about two minutes. Flip and cook the other side until similarly golden brown, about another two minutes. Transfer to a plate. Repeat with the remaining batter, brushing with another tablespoon of oil between batches. (If the pancakes turn too dark, reduce the heat to medium-low. Due to the sweetness of the chocolate, they have a lower smoking point than plain pancakes.) Divide pancakes among four plates, and top with fresh berries. Serve immediately.

ALTERNATE MILK | CASHEW | HAZELNUT |

LUNCH & DINNER ENTRÉES

CASHEW

LASAGNA WITH
BUTTERNUT SQUASH,
SHIITAKE MUSHROOMS,
AND SWISS CHARD

PASTA WITH PUMPKIN-
TOMATO SAUCE WITH
ROSEMARY AND "BACON"

MAC AND CHEESE WITH
TOMATO "BÉCHAMEL"
AND GARLICKY BREAD
CRUMBS

VEGAN PROVENÇAL
QUICHE WITH HEIRLOOM
TOMATOES, OLIVES, AND
FRESH BASIL

CREAMY FETTUCCINE
WITH FIRE-ROASTED
TOMATOES AND BASIL

COCONUT

PUMPKIN AND LENTIL
STEW WITH COCONUT
MILK

MATTAR PANEER
(SPICED PEAS AND TOFU
WITH COCONUT MILK)

DIETARY CATEGORIES: **V** VEGAN VG VEGETARIAN NF NUT-FREE GF GLUTEN-FREE P PALEO

MALAI KOFTA
(VEGETARIAN INDIAN
DUMPLINGS IN SPICED
TOMATO SAUCE)

"BUTTERMILK" "FRIED"
CHICKEN WITH SRIRACHA
HONEY

BELL PEPPER,
MUSHROOM, AND
PINEAPPLE THAI CURRY

CHICKEN AND ROOT
VEGETABLE POTPIE
WITH HERBED BISCUITS

ALMOND

THAI TURKEY BURGERS
WITH LIME AND PEPPER
MAYO

SHEPHERD'S PIE WITH
BEEF, MUSHROOMS, AND
BUTTERNUT SQUASH

SOY

GRILLED ROSEMARY
MUSHROOMS WITH
RED WINE–BALSAMIC
REDUCTION, OVER
POLENTA

LASAGNA WITH BUTTERNUT SQUASH, SHIITAKE MUSHROOMS, AND SWISS CHARD

In this vegetable-rich dish, fresh pasta sheets (available in the refrigerated section) become crispy on the edges. For a vegan variation, opt for dried lasagna sheets, and boil and drain before assembling. • **SERVES 6 TO 8**

2 to 3 tablespoons extra-virgin olive oil, divided

2½ cups small dice butternut squash (about ½ large)

2 scant tablespoons minced garlic (about 4 large cloves)

2 cups sliced (de-stemmed) shiitake mushrooms (about 5 ounces)

5 fresh sage leaves, cut into chiffonade (1 teaspoon)

2 cups thinly sliced Swiss chard leaves, stems removed

1 tablespoon golden or white balsamic vinegar

1 tablespoon red wine vinegar

½ teaspoon kosher salt, divided, plus extra for pasta cooking water

8 grinds black pepper, divided

1 pound fresh lasagna pasta sheets, ideally whole-wheat

2 tablespoons vegan butter

2 tablespoons white whole-wheat flour

1 cup plain unsweetened cashew milk

¼ cup shredded dairy-free mozzarella cheese

2 tablespoons grated dairy-free Parmesan cheese, divided

⅛ teaspoon ground nutmeg

Cooking spray (or more olive oil)

PREHEAT the oven to 400 degrees F. Brush the interior of a 10-inch skillet with 1 tablespoon of the oil, and heat over medium. When warm, add the squash and garlic, and sauté until just tender, about 8 minutes. Add the mushrooms and sage, and sauté until the mushrooms are tender,

about 5 minutes. Stir in the chard, cover, and cook until wilted, about 3 minutes. Stir in both vinegars, half of the salt, and half of the pepper, and simmer for 1 more minute. Remove from the heat, and set aside.

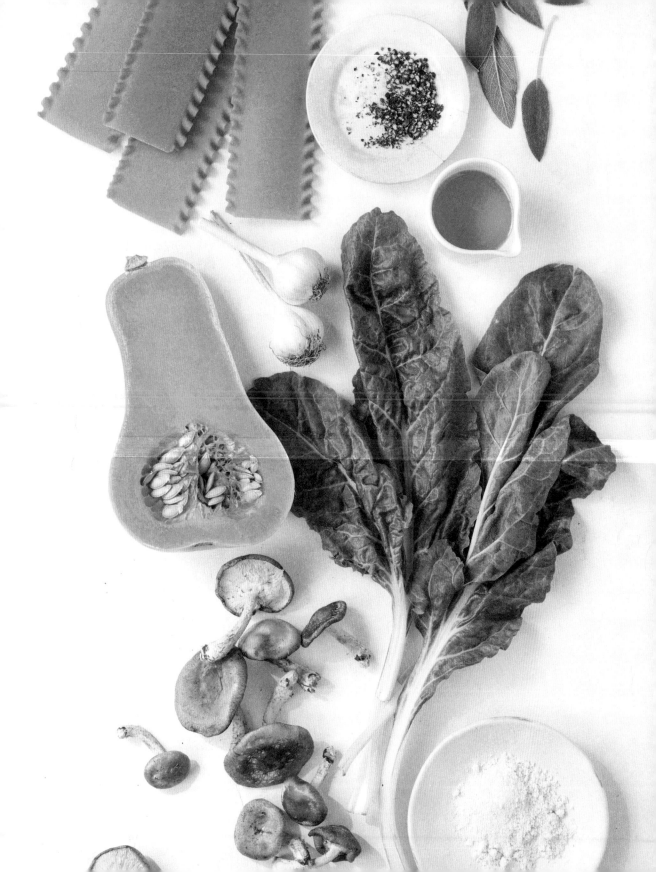

MEANWHILE, fill a medium to large saucepan two-thirds full of salted water, and bring to a boil over high heat. When the water is boiling, carefully add the pasta sheets, stir, and cook until tender, 2 to 3 minutes. Drizzle the remaining oil onto a baking sheet. With tongs, carefully transfer the pasta to the baking sheet, and separate the sheets (if some break slightly, don't worry). Set aside.

WHILE the pasta is boiling, melt the butter over medium heat in a medium to large saucepan. Once the butter is melted, whisk in the flour and cook until it absorbs the butter, about 20 seconds. Whisk in the cashew milk, and raise the heat to medium high. Bring to a simmer and cook, whisking occasionally, until the sauce thickens, about 3 minutes. Remove from the heat, and immediately whisk in the remaining salt and

pepper, the mozzarella, half of the Parmesan, and the nutmeg. Set aside.

GREASE the inside of a roughly 13 x 9-inch baking dish with cooking spray (or more olive oil). Lay one third of the pasta sheets onto the bottom to cover it evenly. Top with half of the vegetable mixture and half of the sauce mixture, spreading evenly with the back of a spoon. Layer on another third of the pasta sheets, and top with the remaining vegetable and sauce mixtures, spreading evenly. Top with the remaining pasta sheets, and sprinkle evenly with the remaining tablespoon of grated Parmesan.

BAKE on the center rack until the pasta turns lightly golden and becomes crisp around the edges, about 40 minutes.

For a gluten-free version, prepare with gluten-free noodles.

ALTERNATE MILK | SOY | RICE |

PASTA WITH PUMPKIN-TOMATO SAUCE WITH ROSEMARY AND "BACON"

Olives, cooked white beans, or braised greens would be nice additions to this dish. Thanks to pumpkin and vegetarian bacon, it's "meaty" and extremely satisfying. Shells, orecchiette, or wheels are an ideal vehicle for this slightly chunky sauce. ● **SERVES 4 (MAKES ABOUT 3 CUPS SAUCE)**

3 cups whole-wheat pasta shells, orecchiette, or wheels

1 tablespoon olive oil

1 cup ¼-inch-dice vegetarian bacon (about a scant ½ pound)

½ cup finely chopped red onion

1 tablespoon finely chopped garlic

1⅓ cups jarred or canned pureed strained tomato (*passata*)

1 cup canned unsweetened pumpkin puree

2 teaspoons minced fresh rosemary leaves

½ teaspoon kosher salt, plus extra for pasta cooking water

5 grinds black pepper

½ cup plain unsweetened cashew milk

FILL a medium-large saucepan two-thirds full of water, and salt generously. Cover and bring to a boil over high heat. Stir in the pasta, and cook following the package directions, stirring occasionally, until *al dente*, about 14 minutes. With a ladle, reserve 3 tablespoons of the pasta water. Drain the pasta in a colander in the sink.

MEANWHILE, add the oil to a Dutch oven or large saucepan, and heat over medium high. When hot, add the "bacon" and cook, stirring occasionally, until golden brown and most of the fat has rendered, about 8 minutes. Pour off most of the fat (leave 2 teaspoons to 1 tablespoon). Add the onion and garlic, and sauté until the onion has softened, 4 to 5 minutes. Add the tomato, pumpkin, rosemary, salt, and pepper, and bring to a boil. Boil for 1 minute. Add the cashew milk, reduce the heat to medium low, and simmer for 3 minutes.

ADD the pasta and the reserved pasta cooking water to the pan with the sauce. With tongs, toss and serve.

For a gluten-free version, prepare with gluten-free pasta.

ALTERNATE MILK | SOY | RICE |

MAC AND CHEESE WITH TOMATO "BÉCHAMEL" AND GARLICKY BREAD CRUMBS

Fire-roasted tomatoes add richness and complexity to this satisfying dairy-free version of a classic. If feeding a crowd, just double the recipe and use a larger baking dish. If you prefer your mac and cheese without any crunch, skip the topping. Instead, just boil the pasta until tender, about eight minutes. Combine with the "béchamel" sauce, and serve immediately (without any baking time). • **SERVES 4 TO 5**

Cooking spray

¼ teaspoon plus ⅛ teaspoon kosher salt, divided, plus extra for the pasta cooking water

2 cups whole-wheat elbow macaroni

3 tablespoons vegan butter, divided

2 tablespoons white whole-wheat flour

1 cup plain unsweetened cashew milk

2 teaspoons Dijon mustard

1 large whole garlic clove plus 1 teaspoon minced garlic, divided

5 grinds black pepper

1 cup shredded vegan Cheddar cheese

¼ cup plus 2 tablespoons canned diced fire-roasted tomatoes, drained

¼ cup whole-wheat panko bread crumbs

PREHEAT the oven to 400 degrees F. Grease a roughly 7 x 7-inch baking dish with cooking spray. Fill a large saucepan two-thirds full of water, salt generously, and bring to a boil over high heat. Once the water is boiling, stir in the pasta, and cook, stirring occasionally, until *al dente* (the minimum time recommended on the packaging), about 7 minutes. Drain the pasta, and set aside.

MEANWHILE, melt 2 tablespoons of the butter in a medium-size, heavy saucepan over medium heat. Once the butter is melted, whisk in the flour, and cook until it is absorbed by the butter, about 30 seconds. Whisk in the cashew milk, mustard, garlic clove, ¼ teaspoon of the salt, and the pepper, and bring to a boil over medium high. As soon as the sauce is thick enough to coat the back of a spoon (about 3 minutes), remove from the heat. Discard the garlic clove. Whisk in the Cheddar and tomatoes, and set aside.

MEANWHILE, place the remaining tablespoon of butter in a medium microwave-safe bowl. Melt in the microwave, about 30 seconds. Stir in the minced garlic, panko, and remaining ⅛ teaspoon salt. Mix well.

POUR the hot cooked pasta into the greased baking dish. With a spatula, scrape in the warm "béchamel" sauce. Mix well in the baking dish. Evenly sprinkle the bread-crumb mixture on top. Bake in the upper third of the oven until the topping becomes golden brown and the mac and cheese crisps up slightly around the edges, about 30 minutes.

ALTERNATE MILK | **SOY** |

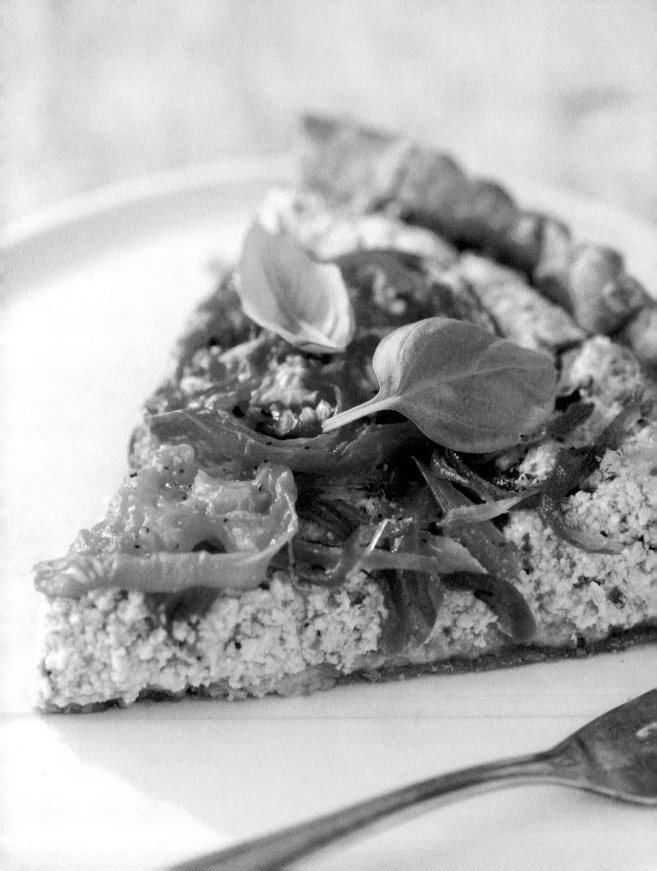

VEGAN PROVENÇAL QUICHE WITH HEIRLOOM TOMATOES, OLIVES, AND FRESH BASIL

This vegan quiche is gorgeous and full of summery tomato-basil-olive flavor. Although it takes about four hours to prepare from start to finish (including chilling time), the dish is well worth it for a festive brunch or summer lunch. • **SERVES 6**

1½ cups plus 3 tablespoons white whole-wheat flour, divided

Scant teaspoon coarse kosher salt, divided

1 stick (8 tablespoons) plus 3 tablespoons vegan butter, chilled and cubed

1 tablespoon flaxseeds, finely ground

6 tablespoons ice-cold water

Cooking spray

1 tablespoon olive oil

2 cups very thin slices red onion (about 2 small)

7 very thin slices heirloom, beefsteak, or hothouse tomato, ideally in 2 to 3 colors

1 12-ounce package plain extra-firm tofu, drained

¼ cup chopped fresh chives

3 tablespoons plain unsweetened cashew milk

2 tablespoons plus 1 teaspoon green olive tapenade or spread (without anchovies), divided

2 teaspoons fresh, strained lemon juice

2 teaspoons cider vinegar

1½ teaspoons agave nectar

1 teaspoon Dijon mustard

4 grinds black pepper

About 8 fresh basil leaves

IN a medium bowl, whisk together 1½ cups plus 1 tablespoon of the flour and ¾ teaspoon of the salt until thoroughly mixed. Add the butter, and crumble together until the mixture forms coarse meal. In a small bowl, whisk together the flaxseeds with the ice-cold water. Add to the flour, and massage the dough until it forms a ball. Wrap in plastic, and flatten into a 1-inch-thick disk. Chill for at least 30 minutes in the fridge.

SPRAY the inside of a 9 or 9½-inch fluted tart pan with a removable bottom with cooking spray. Sprinkle the remaining 2 tablespoons of flour onto a large, clean, cold surface. On this surface, roll the dough into a circle roughly 12 inches in diameter. After each roll, rotate the dough a quarter turn. Transfer the dough circle to the tart pan. Press it into the bottom and sides, rolling the rolling pin over the surface to remove any excess dough (which you can use for patching holes). Cover with plastic wrap and chill for at least 30 minutes. Meanwhile, preheat the oven to 400 degrees F.

PLACE the tart shell on a baking sheet. Spray a large piece of aluminum foil with cooking spray and place the foil, spray side down, onto the dough in the tart pan. Top with dried beans or pie weights. Bake for 20 minutes. Remove from the oven and take off the foil and weights (discard the foil). Use a fork to poke about 15 holes in the bottom of the shell. Return to the oven, and bake until very lightly golden, about another 10 minutes (the crust may shrink a bit).

MEANWHILE, brush the inside of a 10-inch nonstick skillet with oil, and heat over medium. When the oil is warm, add the onions, and sauté for 10 minutes, stirring occasionally. Reduce the heat to low, and continue cooking until the onions are very limp, about another 10 minutes

(watch carefully—you don't want the onions to turn dark brown or black). Place the tomato slices on a large, clean kitchen towel and sprinkle evenly with the remaining salt (a scant ⅛ teaspoon). Cover with another clean kitchen towel and let sit to drain for at least 20 minutes. In a mini food processor, puree the tofu, chives, cashew milk, tapenade, lemon juice, vinegar, agave nectar, mustard, and pepper until smooth, about 1 minute.

REDUCE the oven temperature to 350 degrees F. Pour the custard into the shell, and spread evenly. Sprinkle evenly with the caramelized onions. Overlap the tomato slices around the perimeter of the tart and place one slice in the center.

BAKE until the inside is set (doesn't jiggle), about 45 minutes. Let cool for about 10 minutes, and carefully remove the ring from the tart pan. To do this, lift the tart from the bottom, allowing the ring to fall off. Ideally, chill for at least an hour to allow the filling to further set. Top with the basil.

ALTERNATE MILK | **SOY** |

CREAMY FETTUCCINE WITH FIRE-ROASTED TOMATOES AND BASIL

Tomato, basil, and vegan Parmesan meld beautifully in this kid-friendly dish. If serving six people, prepare twelve ounces of dried pasta; if serving eight, make one pound (the sauce recipe can easily accommodate the latter). I use cheese from the brand GO Veggie! • **SERVES 6 TO 8**

Kosher salt

12 to 16 ounces dried whole-wheat fettuccine

2 tablespoons olive oil

3 tablespoons white whole-wheat flour

3 cups plain unsweetened cashew milk

12 fresh basil leaves, plus another 8 or so for garnish, divided

1 cup shredded vegan mozzarella cheese

¼ cup plus 2 tablespoons canned diced fire-roasted tomatoes, drained

¼ cup plus 2 tablespoons diced seeded fresh tomato (about 1)

¼ cup grated vegan Parmesan cheese

4 grinds black pepper

FILL a medium-large saucepan two-thirds full of water, salt generously, and bring to a boil over high heat. Once the water is boiling, stir in the pasta; cook, following the package directions. Drain and pour the pasta into a very large serving bowl. Cover to keep warm.

MEANWHILE, heat the oil in a medium saucepan over medium heat. When the oil is warm, stir in the flour and cook until it is absorbed, about 30 seconds. Add the cashew milk and 12 basil leaves, and bring to a boil over medium-high heat. Cook, stirring, until the sauce is very smooth and just barely coats the back of a spoon, about 3 minutes (do not let a skin form). Strain into a bowl (dis-

card the basil) and pour the hot sauce back into the hot pot. Whisk in the mozzarella, fire-roasted tomatoes, fresh tomatoes, vegan Parmesan, and black pepper.

POUR the sauce into the serving bowl with the warm pasta. Toss with tongs until the pasta is evenly coated, garnish with fresh basil leaves, and serve immediately. (For a casserole-like dish, opt instead for 3 cups dried whole-wheat elbow macaroni, and cook until al dente. After mixing the cooked pasta with the sauce, pour into a greased 13 x 9-inch baking dish, and bake in a 375 degree F oven until the edges are slightly crisp, about 20 minutes. Garnish and serve.)

ALTERNATE MILK | SOY |

PUMPKIN AND LENTIL STEW WITH COCONUT MILK

Pumpkin puree and light coconut milk add thickness and creaminess to this complex, perfect-for-winter stew. Serve with warm whole-wheat pita or naan bread.

● SERVES 6 (MAKES 8 CUPS)

1 tablespoon safflower oil
1 cup finely chopped red bell pepper
1 cup finely chopped red onion
¾ cup minced celery or leek
½ cup very thinly sliced peeled carrot
1 heaping tablespoon minced jalapeño
1 tablespoon minced garlic
1 tablespoon minced fresh ginger
1 (15-ounce) can unsweetened pumpkin
    puree (about 1½ cups)

1½ cups raw red lentils
1¼ teaspoons coarse kosher salt
4 grinds black pepper
1 quart low-sodium vegetable stock
1 (13.5-ounce) can light coconut milk,
    well shaken
3 tablespoons fresh, strained lime juice
⅓ cup finely chopped fresh cilantro leaves,
    plus another ¼ cup for garnish
2 tablespoons agave nectar

ADD the oil to a medium saucepan, and heat over medium. When warm, add the bell pepper, onion, celery, carrot, jalapeño, garlic, and ginger, and sauté until all of the vegetables are tender, about 15 minutes.

STIR in the pumpkin and lentils, and cook for 1 minute. Add the salt, pepper, stock, coconut milk, and lime juice, and bring to a boil over medium-high heat. Cover, reduce the heat to medium low, and simmer until the lentils are tender, about 35 minutes.

STIR in ⅓ cup of the cilantro and the agave nectar, and ladle into bowls. Garnish with the additional ¼ cup cilantro.

ALTERNATE MILK | CANNED FULL-FAT COCONUT |

MATTAR PANEER
(SPICED PEAS AND TOFU WITH COCONUT MILK)

Tofu stands in for paneer cheese in this Indian-inspired dish. For heat, add some minced chile along with the onion, ginger, and garlic. Prepare some brown rice to serve alongside.

● **SERVES 4**

1 tablespoon coconut oil

½ cup finely chopped red onion

1 tablespoon minced fresh ginger

1 tablespoon minced garlic

½ teaspoon whole yellow mustard seeds

½ teaspoon whole cumin seeds

3 tablespoons tomato paste

1 tablespoon white whole-wheat flour

1 cup canned light coconut milk, well shaken

Scant 2 teaspoons fresh, strained lime juice

1 teaspoon agave nectar

1 pound frozen peas (about 2½ cups), thawed

14 ounces plain extra-firm tofu, cut into
    ½-inch cubes (about 2½ cups)

¾ teaspoon kosher salt

5 grinds black pepper

HEAT the oil in a 10-inch skillet with at least 2-inch-high sides over medium-high heat. Once the oil is hot, add the onion, ginger, garlic, and mustard and cumin seeds, and sauté, stirring occasionally, until the onion is tender, about 6 minutes. Stir in the tomato paste and flour, and whisk until they are incorporated, about

1 minute. Add the coconut milk, lime juice, and agave, and bring to a boil, whisking until smooth, about 3 minutes.

STIR in the peas, tofu, salt, and pepper, and simmer until the sauce thickens and the peas and tofu are coated with the sauce, about 6 minutes. Serve over rice.

ALTERNATE MILK | CANNED FULL-FAT COCONUT | CASHEW |

MALAI KOFTA
(VEGETARIAN INDIAN DUMPLINGS IN SPICED TOMATO SAUCE)

Malai kofta is a traditional North Indian dish, akin to potato dumplings in creamy tomato-based sauce. Coconut milk is not traditional here, but I love the subtle sweetness it imparts. If you're preparing this rich vegan entrée in advance, complete the recipe through straining the sauce. Then reserve the patties and sauce separately. Simmer the patties in the sauce right before serving (if you refrigerate and reheat the patties in the sauce, they can break down and the sauce can form a skin and over-thicken). Serve over rice, and garnish with chopped fresh cilantro leaves. • **SERVES 4**

2 small-medium starchy potatoes, such as Idaho or russet

3½ ounces plain firm tofu, drained

½ cup plus 1 tablespoon almond flour, divided

3 tablespoons plus 2 teaspoons safflower oil, divided

1 teaspoon garam masala, divided

½ teaspoon kosher salt, divided

⅛ teaspoon ground cayenne pepper

3 tablespoons golden raisins or finely chopped dried apricots

1 medium red onion, coarsely chopped (1 heaping cup)

1-inch piece of fresh ginger, coarsely chopped (2 tablespoons)

1 large garlic clove, peeled and coarsely chopped (1 tablespoon)

2 tablespoons plain unsweetened cashew butter

1 tablespoon tomato paste

1½ cups canned light coconut milk, well shaken

1¼ cups jarred or canned pureed strained tomato (*passata*)

1 tablespoon fresh, strained lime juice

1 tablespoon agave nectar

Optional for garnish: finely chopped fresh cilantro leaves

POKE the potatoes all over with a fork, and microwave until very tender, about 18 minutes. Let cool slightly until no longer too hot to handle, then scoop out the flesh (save the skin for another use). Measure out 1¾ cups of the cooked flesh, and add to a food processor. Add the tofu, 3 tablespoons of the almond flour, 1 tablespoon of the oil, ½ teaspoon of the garam masala, ¼ teaspoon of the salt, and the cayenne. Process until the mixture comes together to form a solid mass, about 20 seconds (it will be extremely sticky and stretchy, akin to a dough).

SPRINKLE the remaining 6 tablespoons of almond flour onto a dry surface, such as a clean cutting board. Transfer the potato-tofu ball to the board. Gently knead a few times, working in the remaining almond flour (if the dough is still very sticky, add more almond flour, a tablespoon at a time). Shape into 8 evenly sized patties, and stuff the center of each with raisins (you will use a generous teaspoon per patty).

BRUSH a 10-inch nonstick skillet with 2 tablespoons of the oil, and heat over medium high. When hot, add 4 of the patties, and cook until both sides are golden brown, turning over halfway through, about 6 minutes total. Repeat with the remaining 4 patties. (You will not need more oil and might find that the second batch browns in less time, about 4 minutes total. If you have a large burner and use a 12-inch skillet, you can cook all of the patties in one batch.) Set aside on a plate.

HEAT the remaining 2 teaspoons oil in a medium skillet with at least 2-inch-high sides over medium heat. When warm, add the onion, ginger, garlic, the remaining ½ teaspoon garam masala, and the remaining ¼ teaspoon salt. Sauté until the onion has softened, about 5 minutes. Add the cashew butter and tomato paste, and cook for about 3 minutes, stirring occasionally. Add the coconut milk, pureed tomatoes, lime juice, and agave nectar, and bring to a boil over medium-high heat. Boil until thick enough to just coat the back of a spoon, about 3 minutes.

PLACE a fine or coarse strainer over a large bowl, and carefully pour the sauce through (discard the solids and scrape any extra sauce from the bottom of the strainer). Pour the sauce back into the skillet (carefully wipe it out first), and bring to a low simmer over medium heat. Once simmering, add the patties; cover; and cook on medium low for 3 minutes. Carefully flip over the patties; recover the pan; and continue cooking until they puff up slightly, another 2 to 3 minutes. Serve, ladling 2 patties and one quarter of the sauce into each serving bowl.

ALTERNATE MILK | CANNED FULL-FAT COCONUT MILK |

BELL PEPPER, MUSHROOM, AND PINEAPPLE THAI CURRY

Vegetables star in this colorful Thai-inspired stew. If you're vegetarian or vegan, omit the fish sauce; just substitute an extra two teaspoons of low-sodium soy sauce. To add protein, stir in one package of extra-firm tofu, drained and cut into half-inch cubes. • **SERVES 4 TO 6**

1 (13.5-ounce) can light coconut milk, well shaken (about 1¾ cups)

2 tablespoons fresh, strained lime juice

2 tablespoons low-sodium tamari soy sauce

2 tablespoons agave nectar

1 tablespoon creamy peanut butter

1 tablespoon cornstarch

2 teaspoons fish sauce

2 tablespoons safflower oil, divided

Scant ½ cup finely chopped red onion (½ small)

Scant tablespoon minced garlic

Scant tablespoon minced fresh ginger

Scant tablespoon minced jalapeño

Heaping ½ cup ½-inch-dice red bell pepper (seeds and membranes removed)

Heaping ½ cup ½-inch-dice yellow bell pepper (seeds and membranes removed)

3 cups quartered white button or cremini mushrooms (about 10 ounces)

3 cups ½-inch-dice pineapple

4 cups trimmed snow peas

2 to 3 cups cooked short-grain brown rice, for serving

IN a medium bowl, whisk together the first seven ingredients until as smooth as possible. Set aside.

PLACE a large wok (preferably cast iron) over high heat, and let heat until hot, about 3 minutes. (If using a nonstick wok, brush with oil before heating, and then cook over medium high.) Brush with 1 tablespoon of the oil. When hot, add the onion, garlic, ginger, and jalapeño, and sauté until aromatic, about 1 minute. Add the bell peppers and mushrooms, and sauté until both are tender, about 8 minutes, adding the remaining tablespoon of oil when the pan becomes dry.

STIR in all of the sauce you made in the first step, along with the pineapple, and bring to a gentle simmer. Stir in the snow peas. Cover and simmer over medium low until the snow peas are crisp-tender and still bright green and the sauce has thickened, about 4 minutes. Ladle immediately over rice in shallow bowls.

Kosher if using kosher fish sauce

ALTERNATE MILK | **CANNED FULL-FAT COCONUT MILK** |

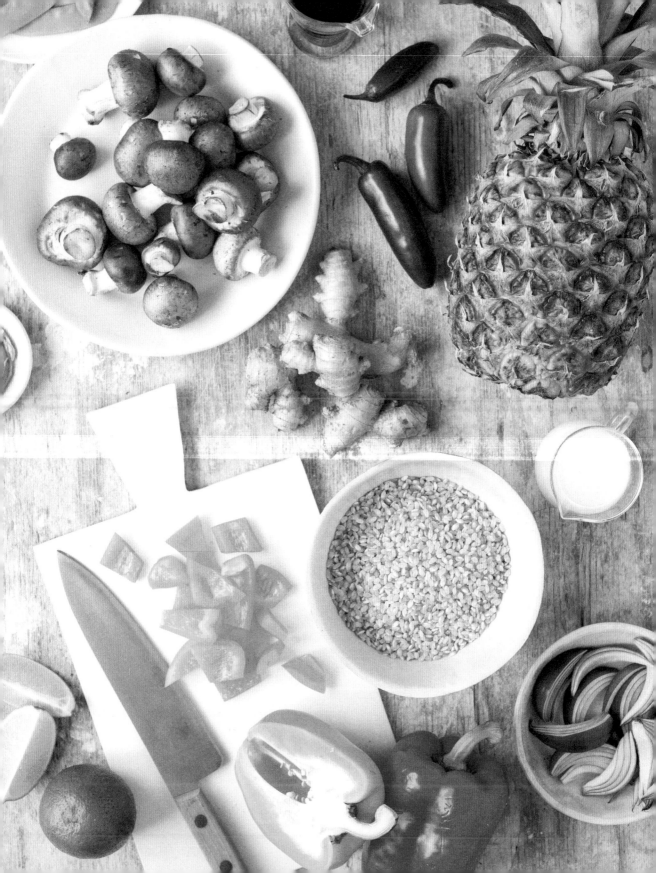

THAI TURKEY BURGERS WITH LIME AND PEPPER MAYO

These turkey burgers are full of flavor. If using ground thigh meat, slightly reduce the quantity of mayo. • **SERVES 4**

½ cup plain whole-wheat bread crumbs

3 tablespoons plain unsweetened coconut milk beverage (not canned)

3 tablespoons finely chopped fresh cilantro leaves

2 tablespoons thinly sliced green onion

¼ cup plus 2 tablespoons mayonnaise, divided

1 tablespoon minced peeled trimmed lemongrass

1 tablespoon minced fresh ginger

1 tablespoon agave nectar

1 tablespoon low-sodium tamari soy sauce

2 teaspoons minced jalapeño

1 teaspoon fish sauce

1½ teaspoons freshly grated lime zest, divided

1 pound ground turkey breast

2 teaspoons safflower oil

5 grinds black pepper

For serving: 4 toasted split whole-wheat burger buns, 4 slices tomato, 4 very thin slices red onion, and 4 romaine leaves

IN a large bowl, stir together the first four ingredients, 2 tablespoons of the mayonnaise, the lemongrass, ginger, agave nectar, soy sauce, jalapeño, fish sauce, and 1 teaspoon of the zest. Add the turkey, and massage until well mixed. Shape into four 1-inch-thick patties, and indent each one in the center.

BRUSH the inside of a 10-inch nonstick skillet with the oil, and heat over medium high. When hot, add the patties, and cook until the first side is golden brown, 4 minutes. Flip with a spatula, and cook until the other side is also golden brown, about another 4 minutes. Reduce the heat to medium low, and continue cooking until the patties are cooked in the center, about another 2 minutes (do not let the patties get too dark).

MEANWHILE, in a small bowl, stir together the remaining ¼ cup mayonnaise, the remaining ½ teaspoon zest, and the black pepper.

ATOP each bun half, place a romaine leaf. Top with a turkey patty, tomato slice, red onion slice, and dollop of mayonnaise. Serve immediately.

For a gluten-free version, use gluten-free bread crumbs and buns.

ALTERNATE MILK | CASHEW | SOY |

GRILLED ROSEMARY MUSHROOMS WITH RED WINE–BALSAMIC REDUCTION, OVER POLENTA

This elegant, meaty yet meat-free dish features polenta, made creamy thanks to soy milk. When scraping the gills from the underside of the mushroom caps, be sure to preserve their round shape. • **SERVES 4**

2 cups plain unsweetened soy milk

1 teaspoon kosher salt, divided

12 grinds black pepper, divided

1 cup uncooked polenta

4 tablespoons vegan butter, divided

½ cup medium- to full-bodied fruity red wine

¼ cup plus 1 tablespoon balsamic vinegar, divided

¼ cup extra-virgin olive oil

1 tablespoon finely chopped fresh rosemary leaves

3 medium garlic cloves, coarsely chopped

14 ounces portobello mushroom caps (4 large caps), stems trimmed and gills scraped out

1 tablespoon safflower oil

ADD the soy milk, 2 cups water, ½ teaspoon of the salt, and 4 grinds of the pepper to a medium-large saucepan. Bring to a boil over medium-high heat. Whisk in the polenta, and cook, stirring, until it thickens and begins to sputter, about 3 minutes. Reduce the heat to low, and cook, stirring every 5 to 10 minutes, until the polenta becomes tender, about 35 minutes. Stir in 2 tablespoons of the vegan butter. (You should have 3 cups polenta.)

MEANWHILE, add the wine and ¼ cup of the vinegar to a small saucepan, and bring to a boil over medium-high heat. Reduce the heat to medium, and simmer until the mixture cooks down to a scant ⅓ cup and coats the back of a spoon, about 12 minutes. Stir in the remaining 2 tablespoons vegan butter (you should have ¼ cup sauce).

WHILE the sauce is reducing, in a medium-large bowl, stir together the olive oil, the remaining tablespoon of vinegar, the rosemary, and the garlic. Add the mushrooms, and marinate for 15 minutes, turning to coat (rub the marinade into the undersides of the caps).

GENTLY pat the mushrooms dry, and season both sides evenly with the remaining 8 grinds of pepper and ½ teaspoon salt. Heat a grill pan over medium-high heat, and brush with the safflower oil. When hot, add the mushrooms, and grill, turning over halfway through, until they acquire grill marks and collapse a bit, about 7 minutes total.

ONTO each plate, scoop one quarter of the polenta, and place a mushroom cap on top. Drizzle each portion with 1 tablespoon of the sauce, and serve.

ALTERNATE MILK | CASHEW | RICE |

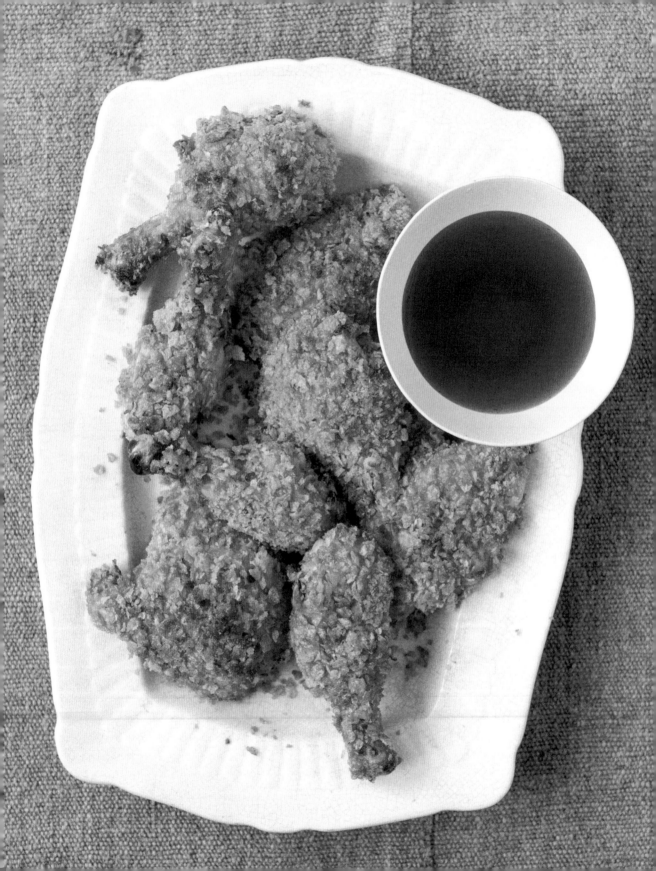

"BUTTERMILK" "FRIED" CHICKEN WITH SRIRACHA HONEY

Baked and seasoned with Sriracha and lime, this lighter "fried" chicken has a slightly Asian feel. Note that it takes at least 2 hours to marinate, so plan ahead. Crush the cornflakes by placing them in a plastic bag and sealing; bash with a rolling pin or meat mallet or the bottom of a heavy pot. For maximum crispiness, serve immediately after baking. • **SERVES 4**

2 cups plain unsweetened soy milk

2 tablespoons fresh, strained lime juice

3 tablespoons Sriracha sauce, divided

1½ tablespoons crushed chopped garlic

1¼ teaspoons coarse kosher salt, divided

18 grinds black pepper, divided

About 2¾ pounds bone-in chicken thighs and drumsticks (about 4 thighs and 5 drumsticks), skin removed

Cooking spray

4 cups cornflake cereal, crushed (about 1¼ cups)

4 tablespoons vegan butter, melted

¼ cup honey

IN a large bowl, whisk together the soy milk and lime juice, and let sit for 10 minutes. Add 2 tablespoons of the Sriracha, the garlic, ½ teaspoon of the salt, and 10 grinds of the pepper, and whisk again. Add the chicken, covering with the marinade. Cover and chill for at least 2 hours or overnight.

WHEN ready to bake the chicken, preheat the oven to 400 degrees F, and place an oven rack in the second highest position. Place a wire rack on top of a rimmed baking sheet, and spray the wire rack with cooking spray.

IN a medium bowl, whisk together the crushed cornflakes with the remaining ¾ teaspoon salt and 8 grinds of pepper. One at a time, remove a piece of chicken from the marinade, shaking off the liquid. Discard the marinade. Dredge both sides in the seasoned cornflakes, and transfer to the rack. Repeat with the remaining chicken and cornflakes. Evenly drizzle the melted vegan butter over the chicken.

BAKE until the outside of the chicken is golden brown and the meat is 165 degrees F when poked with a meat thermometer (not touching bone), about 40 minutes. (Do not turn over the chicken.) Let cool for 5 minutes.

MEANWHILE, add the remaining tablespoon Sriracha plus the honey to a small saucepan, and bring to a simmer over medium heat. Turn off the heat and keep at room temperature. Gently transfer the chicken to plates. Serve with the Sriracha honey on the side for dipping.

Kosher if made with kosher chicken

ALTERNATE MILK | COCONUT | CASHEW |

CHICKEN AND ROOT VEGETABLE POTPIE WITH HERBED BISCUITS

This comforting autumnal dish involves several steps, but is well worth it. For a vegetarian variation, try meat-free sausage with sage. • **SERVES 4 TO 6**

3 cups plain unsweetened soy milk, divided

1 tablespoon fresh, strained lemon juice

3 cups plus 3 tablespoons white whole-wheat flour, divided

1 tablespoon Sucanat or brown sugar

1 tablespoon baking powder

2 teaspoons minced fresh rosemary leaves

1½ teaspoons plus ⅛ teaspoon kosher salt, divided

½ teaspoon baking soda

7½ tablespoons vegan butter, very cold, divided

About 1⅔ pounds (26 ounces) boneless, skinless chicken thighs, cut into 1-inch cubes

1 tablespoon vegetable oil

1 cup coarsely chopped red onion (about 1)

1 cup coarsely chopped green apple (about 1)

1 cup coarsely chopped parsnip (about 2)

1 cup coarsely chopped carrot (about 2)

1 cup thinly sliced leek (white and light green parts only), rinsed and drained (about ½ large leek)

2 tablespoons minced garlic

1 tablespoon minced fresh sage leaves

5 grinds black pepper

¼ cup apple juice

MAKE THE BISCUITS: Preheat the oven to 450 degrees F. In a small-medium bowl, mix 1 cup of the soy milk and all of the lemon juice, and let sit for 10 minutes. Meanwhile, in a large bowl, whisk together 2 cups plus 2 tablespoons of the flour, the Sucanat, baking powder, rosemary, ½ teaspoon plus ⅛ teaspoon of the salt, and the baking soda until well blended. Cut 5 tablespoons of the butter into small cubes, and add to the flour mixture. Using a pastry blender or your fingers, crumble the butter into the flour until it forms coarse meal. Pour in the milk mixture, and gently knead in the bowl just until a smooth dough forms (avoid overworking).

TRANSFER the dough to a cold clean surface, and pat into a 4 x 4-inch rectangle 1 inch thick. With a sharp 2-inch biscuit cutter, cut into about 8 rounds, and transfer to a baking sheet. The biscuits should be spaced 1 inch apart. Meanwhile, melt ½ tablespoon of the butter in the microwave, about 25 seconds. Brush on top of the biscuits.

IMMEDIATELY transfer to the oven, and bake on the middle rack until golden brown and cooked through, about 12 minutes.

MEANWHILE, MAKE THE FILLING: In a medium-large bowl, use tongs to toss the chicken with the remaining 5 tablespoons of flour. Heat the remaining 2 tablespoons butter with the oil in a Dutch oven over medium-high heat. Once the butter has melted, add the chicken, and cook until golden brown and mostly cooked, turning over halfway through, 8 to 10 minutes. Transfer to a plate or bowl.

TO the hot pot, add the onion, apple, parsnip, carrot, leek, garlic, sage, black pepper, and the remaining teaspoon of salt. Sauté, stirring occasionally, until the carrot and parsnip are two-thirds cooked through, about 8 minutes. Add the juice and remaining 2 cups soy milk, and bring to a full boil. Stir back in the chicken and any juices from the plate.

COVER and reduce the heat to medium low. Simmer until the chicken is fully cooked and the sauce has thickened (the parsnip will break down to further thicken the sauce), about 8 minutes. Stir the sauce until smooth.

ASSEMBLE THE POTPIE: For a family-style presentation, ladle the chicken-vegetable-sauce mixture into a 13 x 9-inch baking dish. Top evenly with the 8 warm biscuits. (For individual presentations, ladle the filling into 6 large ramekins, and top each one with one biscuit—you'll have two biscuits left over.)

Kosher if you use kosher chicken

ALTERNATE MILK | CASHEW |

SHEPHERD'S PIE WITH BEEF, MUSHROOMS, AND BUTTERNUT SQUASH

Fresh and dried mushrooms add complexity to this shepherd's pie. To prepare your own porcini powder, grind about two tablespoons of dried porcini mushrooms in a spice grinder or cleaned coffee grinder until powdery, about one minute. Be sure to cut the parsnips into small pieces, as they take a while to cook. If you don't have butternut squash, try pumpkin or carrots. For a vegan version, use crumbled meat-free sausage, such as Field Roast.

● SERVES 6 TO 8

3 russet or Idaho potatoes

¾ cup plain unsweetened almond milk, at room temperature

¼ cup (4 tablespoons) vegan butter, at room temperature

1 tablespoon plus 1 teaspoon ground dried porcini mushroom (porcini powder; see above note)

1 teaspoon kosher salt, divided

10 grinds black pepper, divided

1 tablespoon olive oil

1 pound ground beef chuck

2 cups small dice cremini mushrooms (about 6 ounces)

1¼ cups small dice butternut squash

¾ cup small dice parsnip

¾ cup finely chopped red onion

1 tablespoon finely chopped garlic

3 tablespoons tomato paste

1 tablespoon finely chopped fresh sage leaves

1 tablespoon finely chopped fresh oregano leaves

¾ teaspoon ground nutmeg

Cooking spray

PREHEAT the oven to 375 degrees F. Poke the potatoes several times, and microwave on high until extremely tender, about 20 minutes. When no longer too hot to handle, split in half, and scoop 4 cups of their flesh into a medium-large bowl (save the skins for another use). Add the almond milk, vegan butter, ground porcini, ½ teaspoon of the salt, and half of the pepper, and mash with a potato masher until smooth.

MEANWHILE, brush the inside of a 10-inch non-stick skillet with 2-inch-high sides with the oil, and heat over medium high. When warm, add the beef, and cook, breaking it up with a wooden spoon, until no longer pink, about 8 minutes. Transfer to a plate. To the hot pan, add the cremini mushrooms, squash, parsnip, onion, and garlic. Sauté, stirring occasionally, until all of the vegetables are soft, about 10 minutes (if necessary, add a couple tablespoons of water to help the parsnips become tender).

POUR the vegetables into a medium-large mixing bowl, and add the meat, tomato paste, sage, oregano, nutmeg, and remaining ½ teaspoon salt, and the remaining 5 grinds pepper. Mix well.

SPRAY the inside of an 8 x 8-inch baking dish with cooking spray. Pour in the meat-vegetable filling. Top with the potato mixture, and spread evenly. Bake on the middle rack of the oven until the potatoes become lightly golden and slightly crispy on the sides, about 30 minutes.

Kosher if you use kosher meat

ALTERNATE MILK | **SOY** | RICE |

SOUPS, SIDES, SAUCES & DRESSINGS

SOUPS

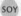

CASHEW

VICHYSSOISE WITH
FENNEL

CREAMY MUSHROOM
SOUP WITH CHIVES

SOY

SOUTHWESTERN
CORN CHOWDER WITH
"BACON" AND BELL
PEPPER

COCONUT

COCONUT CARROT
SOUP WITH
LEMONGRASS AND LIME

SIDES

HAZELNUT

PARSNIP PUREE WITH
HAZELNUTS AND SAGE

CASHEW

VEGAN "CREAMED"
SPINACH WITH GARLIC
AND NUTMEG

 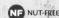

MASHED SWEET POTATOES
WITH PINEAPPLE AND
SRIRACHA

CASHEW

TOMATO "CREAM" SAUCE
WITH OREGANO AND
CHILE FLAKES

MASHED CAULIFLOWER
WITH "BROWN BUTTER"
AND SAGE

COCONUT

MISO-GINGER DRESSING

SOY

MASHED POTATOES
WITH GARLIC AND
CHIVES

RICE

MANGO-LIME DRESSING

SAUCES AND DRESSINGS

SOY

BEET CREAM

TAHINI AND MINT
DRESSING

CREAMY BASIL AND
CHIVE DRESSING

VICHYSSOISE WITH FENNEL

A chilled French soup, vichyssoise includes leeks and potatoes; here, I've added fennel for anise notes. To rinse the leeks, slice and transfer to a large bowl full of water. Swish around until no dirt remains, replacing the water a couple of times if necessary, then drain.

● **MAKES 8 SCANT CUPS (ABOUT 4 SERVINGS)**

2 tablespoons vegan butter

2 leeks, trimmed, halved, sliced, and rinsed (2 cups)

½ large fennel bulb, trimmed, cored, and coarsely chopped (1 cup)

1 starchy medium-large potato, such as Idaho or russet, peeled and thinly sliced (2 scant cups)

2 tablespoons white whole-wheat flour

2½ cups low-sodium vegetable stock

½ teaspoon kosher salt

4 grinds black pepper

1 cup plain unflavored cashew milk

¼ cup minced fresh chives

ADD the butter to a Dutch oven, and melt over medium heat. Once the butter is melted, add the leeks and fennel, cover, and cook until tender, about 8 minutes.

ADD the potato and flour, and stir until the flour is absorbed, about a minute. Add the stock, salt, and pepper, and bring to a boil over high heat.

Cover and reduce the heat to medium low to low. Simmer until the potato is very tender, about 30 minutes.

CAREFULLY transfer mixture to a food processor or blender; add the cashew milk; and puree until very smooth, about 45 seconds. Chill until cold. Serve, garnishing with the chives.

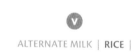

ALTERNATE MILK | RICE |

CREAMY MUSHROOM SOUP WITH CHIVES

For a colder weather version, use red wine instead of lemon juice, and minced fresh thyme or rosemary instead of chives. • **SERVES 4 (MAKES ABOUT 5 CUPS)**

3 tablespoons vegan butter, divided

1 tablespoon olive oil

1 cup finely chopped red onion

1 tablespoon finely chopped garlic

4 cups sliced white button mushrooms (10 ounces)

1 quart vegetable stock

¼ cup dried wild mushrooms, such as porcini

2 tablespoons fresh, strained lemon juice

¼ teaspoon kosher salt

8 grinds black pepper

½ cup plain unsweetened cashew milk, at room temperature

¼ cup minced fresh chives, plus additional 2 teaspoons for garnish, if desired

MELT 1 tablespoon of the vegan butter with the oil over medium heat in a Dutch oven or medium saucepan. Add the onion and garlic, and sauté until the onion has softened, 3 or 4 minutes. Add the button mushrooms, and sauté until softened, about 3 minutes. Add the stock, dried mushrooms, lemon juice, salt, and pepper, and raise the heat to medium high. Bring to a boil, then cover and simmer over low heat for 20 minutes.

STIR in the cashew milk, the remaining 2 tablespoons vegan butter, and the chives. Puree with an immersion blender, blender, or food processor until smooth. Serve warm, garnishing with extra chives.

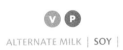

ALTERNATE MILK | **SOY** |

SOUTHWESTERN CORN CHOWDER WITH "BACON" AND BELL PEPPER

Corn cobs (stripped of their kernels) and diced potatoes thicken the broth of this rich and creamy soup. Try topping with diced avocado and pico de gallo or salsa. Make sure to strip all of the silk from the corn. • **MAKES ABOUT 7½ CUPS (ABOUT 4 SERVINGS)**

1 tablespoon safflower oil

5 strips vegetarian bacon (4 to 5 ounces), finely chopped (1 scant cup)

1 cup finely chopped red bell pepper (about 1)

¾ cup finely chopped red onion (about 1 small)

1 teaspoon minced jalapeño

4 ears corn, kernels removed (about 3 cups), cobs reserved

½ teaspoon ground cumin

½ teaspoon kosher salt

5 cups plain unsweetened soy milk

1 cup small dice peeled starchy potato, such as russet (about 1 small)

½ cup minced fresh chives

ADD the oil to a Dutch oven, and heat over medium high. When hot, add the "bacon" and cook, stirring occasionally, until it becomes golden brown and the fat renders, about 8 minutes. Add the bell pepper, onion, and jalapeño, and sauté until relatively soft, 4 minutes. Add the corn kernels (not the cobs), cumin, and salt, and sauté until the corn is tender, about 2 minutes. Add the soy milk and stripped cobs, and bring to a boil.

COVER and reduce the heat to low; simmer for 25 minutes. Stir in the potato, re-cover, and simmer until the liquid is thick and the potato is tender, about another 5 minutes. Remove and discard the cobs, stir the soup well to mix in any errant starch, and stir in the chives. Ladle into bowls, and serve immediately.

For a gluten-free version, prepare with gluten-free bacon.

ALTERNATE MILK | RICE | CASHEW |

COCONUT CARROT SOUP WITH LEMONGRASS AND LIME

This velvety, sweet, and slightly spicy orange soup was inspired by Thai cuisine. Serve it as a starter before spiced sautéed tofu stir-fry, or the Thai turkey burgers on page 40.

● **MAKES ABOUT 7½ CUPS**

1 tablespoon safflower or coconut oil

1 cup finely chopped red onion

1½ tablespoons finely chopped jalapeño (seeds and membrane removed)

1 heaping tablespoon peeled trimmed lemongrass, minced

1 tablespoon finely chopped fresh ginger

4 cups ¼-thick-slices carrot (about 4 large)

2 tablespoons tomato paste

1 quart vegetable broth or stock

1 (14-ounce) can (full-fat) coconut milk (about 1¾ cups), well shaken

2 scant tablespoons fresh, strained lime juice

1 tablespoon agave nectar

¼ teaspoon kosher salt

Optional for serving: finely chopped fresh cilantro leaves

HEAT the oil in a Dutch oven or medium-large saucepan over medium heat. When warm, add the onion, jalapeño, lemongrass, and ginger, and sauté until softened, 3 to 4 minutes. Add the carrots, and sauté for 3 minutes. Stir in the tomato paste, and cook for 1 minute. Add the broth, coconut milk, lime juice, agave nectar, and salt, and bring to a boil over medium-high heat.

COVER and simmer over low heat until the carrots are very tender, about 30 minutes. Puree with an immersion blender, blender, or food processor until very smooth (make sure no chunks remain). Ladle into bowls and serve, garnishing with the cilantro.

ALTERNATE MILK | CANNED LIGHT COCONUT MILK |

PARSNIP PUREE WITH HAZELNUTS AND SAGE

Sweet and nutty hazelnut milk complements the flavor of parsnips. If you use unsweetened hazelnut milk, add about 2 teaspoons agave nectar. To chiffonade sage leaves, stack in one pile; roll up; and thinly slice. To remove the skins from hazelnuts, toast on a baking sheet in a 350-degree oven for ten minutes. Transfer to a kitchen towel; bundle up; and rub until the papery skins fall off. For ease, just warm the milk in the microwave.

● **MAKES 2 CUPS (4 SERVINGS)**

1 pound fresh parsnips (5 to 6), trimmed, peeled, and thinly sliced (3¼ cups)
½ cup plain hazelnut milk (sweetened), warmed
2 tablespoons plus 1 teaspoon extra-virgin olive oil, divided

8 fresh sage leaves, cut in chiffonade (1 tablespoon)
¼ teaspoon plus ⅛ teaspoon kosher salt
5 grinds black pepper
¼ cup hazelnuts, toasted and skins rubbed off, nuts finely chopped

INSERT a steamer basket in a medium saucepan. Add 2 inches of water, and bring to a boil over medium-high heat. Place the parsnips in the basket, cover, and steam until very tender, about 20 minutes.

IMMEDIATELY transfer to the bowl of a food processor. Add the hazelnut milk, 2 tablespoons of the oil, the sage, salt, and pepper, and puree until smooth, about 30 seconds.

TRANSFER to a bowl, top with the nuts, and drizzle with the remaining teaspoon of oil.

ALTERNATE MILK | PLAIN SWEETENED ALMOND | QUINOA |

VEGAN "CREAMED" SPINACH WITH GARLIC AND NUTMEG

I love to spoon this delicious creamed spinach over baked potatoes. It's also delicious as a sandwich spread or in lasagna. If using fresh spinach, you'll need about six cups of chopped leaves (stems removed). Cook the spinach until wilted before adding the cashew milk sauce.

● **SERVES 4 (MAKES 2½ CUPS)**

2 tablespoons vegan butter

2 tablespoons all-purpose white or whole-wheat flour

1 cup plain unsweetened cashew milk

¼ teaspoon kosher salt

⅛ teaspoon black pepper

¹⁄₁₆ teaspoon ground nutmeg

¼ cup finely grated vegan Parmesan cheese, such as Go Veggie!

2 teaspoons olive oil

1 tablespoon minced garlic

1-pound bag frozen spinach, thawed, drained, and squeezed dry

MELT the butter in a small, heavy saucepan over medium heat. Once the butter is melted, whisk in the flour, and cook until it is absorbed into the butter, about 20 seconds. Whisk in the milk, salt, pepper, and nutmeg, and raise the heat to medium high. Bring to a simmer, whisking occasionally. Simmer until it thickens enough to coat the back of a spoon (about 2 minutes). Off of the heat, immediately whisk in the Parmesan, and set aside.

MEANWHILE, brush the interior of a 10-inch non-stick skillet with the oil, and heat over medium. Once warm, add the garlic and sauté until aromatic, about 1 minute (do not let brown). Add the spinach, and cook, stirring, for about 1 minute. Scrape the cream mixture into the skillet. Stir well, remove from the heat, and serve immediately.

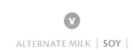

ALTERNATE MILK | SOY |

MASHED SWEET POTATOES WITH PINEAPPLE AND SRIRACHA

Try this puree alongside Asian-inspired mains, such as tofu stir-fry or roast duck. For children, omit the spicy Sriracha sauce. • **MAKES ABOUT 2 SERVINGS (1 CUP)**

2 small sweet potatoes or yams
¼ cup cubed ripe fresh pineapple
¼ cup plain unsweetened cashew milk

1 tablespoon vegan butter
½ teaspoon Sriracha sauce
¼ teaspoon kosher salt

POKE the sweet potatoes all over with a fork, and microwave until very tender, about 12 minutes.

WHEN cool enough to handle, but still warm, scoop out the flesh (you should yield about ¾ cup). Transfer to the bowl of a food processor. Add the remaining ingredients, and puree until very smooth, about 40 seconds.

ALTERNATE MILK | ALMOND | COCONUT (CANNED OR BEVERAGE) |

MASHED CAULIFLOWER WITH "BROWN BUTTER" AND SAGE

Browning the vegan butter adds a toasted hazelnut flavor. Serve this side, similar in consistency to mashed potatoes, with sweet potato or mushroom lasagna or seared fish or tofu. ● **MAKES ABOUT 3 CUPS**

6 cups cauliflower florets (about 1 medium head)
4 tablespoons vegan butter
½ cup plain unsweetened cashew or hazelnut milk, warm or at room temperature

1½ tablespoons minced fresh sage leaves
½ teaspoon kosher salt
8 grinds black pepper

STEAM the cauliflower until very tender, about 10 minutes (poke with a fork to check; it should go in easily). Reserve ¼ cup of the hot water.

MEANWHILE, add the vegan butter to a small sauté pan, and heat over medium. Cook until the butter fully melts and turns a very light

golden brown color, about 8 minutes (watch carefully).

POUR into a bowl. Add the steamed cauliflower and remaining ingredients, including the reserved hot water. Puree with an immersion blender, blender, or food processor until smooth.

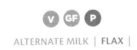

ALTERNATE MILK | **FLAX** |

MASHED POTATOES WITH GARLIC AND CHIVES

Feel free to double this recipe for holiday meals. Just use a Dutch oven or large saucepan.

● **MAKES ABOUT 2½ CUPS**

3¼ cups ½-inch dice peeled russet or Idaho
  potato (about 2 medium)
1½ cups plain unsweetened soy milk
2 medium garlic cloves, peeled and crushed
½ teaspoon kosher salt

4 grinds black pepper
3 tablespoons minced fresh chives
2 tablespoons vegan butter, melted
1 tablespoon extra-virgin olive oil

ADD the potatoes, soy milk, garlic, salt, and pepper to a deep medium-large saucepan, and bring to a boil over medium-high heat.

REDUCE the heat to low, cover, and simmer until the potatoes are very tender, about 15 minutes (the milk might boil over slightly). Add the chives, vegan butter, and oil, and mash with a potato masher until smooth and creamy.

ALTERNATE MILK | CASHEW | FLAX |

BEET CREAM

This smooth pink-purple cream is sweet and earthy. Try serving it as a sauce with grilled mushrooms, tofu, tempeh, or steak. Beet cream is also delicious on smoked salmon and cucumber sandwiches, or even as a dip with potato chips. For ease, purchase precooked beets. • **MAKES ABOUT 3½ CUPS**

1 pound plain silken tofu (about 2 cups)

About 7 small, peeled roasted beets (about 13 ounces, or 2 cups)

2 tablespoons plain unsweetened soy milk

1 tablespoon fresh, strained lemon juice

2 teaspoons agave nectar

½ teaspoon coarse kosher salt

8 grinds black pepper

ADD all of the ingredients to a food processor, and puree until smooth, about 1½ minutes.

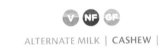

ALTERNATE MILK | **CASHEW** |

TAHINI AND MINT DRESSING

Nutty and creamy, this dressing tastes a bit like hummus. Toss it with tomatoes, cucumber, kale or romaine, toasted whole-wheat pita wedges, pomegranate seeds, and cooked chickpeas. Feel free to add some cumin, coriander, and cayenne. ● **MAKES ABOUT ¾ CUP**

1 very large garlic clove
⅓ cup packed fresh mint leaves
¼ cup plain unsweetened soy milk
3 tablespoons extra-virgin olive oil
2 tablespoons tahini (well stirred)

2 tablespoons fresh, strained lemon juice
2 teaspoons agave nectar
¼ teaspoon kosher salt
3 grinds black pepper

ADD the garlic to the bowl of a mini food processor, and process until finely chopped, about 10 seconds. Add the remaining ingredients, and process until smooth, about 40 seconds.

ALTERNATE MILK | CASHEW | ALMOND |

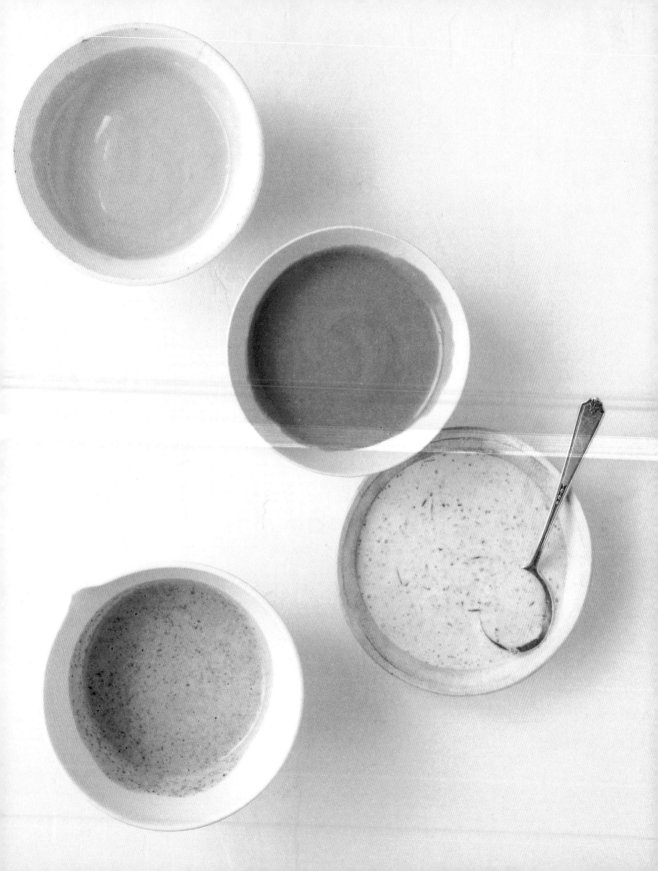

CREAMY BASIL AND CHIVE DRESSING

Drizzle this creamy dressing over a tomato and avocado salad. Also try serving as a dip for vegetables. Feel free to vary the herbs; for instance, swapping in fresh parsley for half of the chives. To reduce the fat, use silken tofu for a portion of the sour cream. • **MAKES 2¼ CUPS**

1 cup plain unsweetened soy milk
2 tablespoons plus 1 teaspoon fresh, strained
    lemon juice
½ cup dairy-free sour cream
3 tablespoons mayonnaise, vegan or
    traditional
½ cup chopped fresh basil leaves

½ cup chopped fresh chives
1 garlic clove
2 teaspoons red wine vinegar
2 teaspoons agave nectar
1½ teaspoons Dijon mustard
¼ teaspoon kosher salt
5 grinds black pepper

IN a small bowl, stir together the soy milk and lemon juice, and let sit for 10 minutes. Add,

along with the remaining ingredients, to a food processor. Blend until smooth, about 1 minute.

ALTERNATE MILK | RICE | CASHEW |

TOMATO "CREAM" SAUCE WITH OREGANO AND CHILE FLAKES

Treat this slightly spicy sauce like a marinara, and use it for eggplant and chicken Parmesan, and pasta. ● **MAKES ABOUT 1¾ CUPS**

2 teaspoons olive oil

1½ tablespoons finely chopped garlic

3 cups jarred or canned pureed strained tomato (*passata*)

1 tablespoon red wine vinegar

½ teaspoon kosher salt

¼ teaspoon dried oregano

⅛ teaspoon crushed red chile flakes

5 grinds black pepper

½ cup plain unsweetened cashew milk

2 tablespoons vegan butter

HEAT the oil in a medium-large saucepan over medium heat. When warm, add the garlic, and sauté until aromatic, about 1 minute. Add the tomatoes, vinegar, salt, oregano, chile flakes, and black pepper, and bring to a boil over medium-high heat.

COVER and reduce the heat to medium low. Simmer until thickened and reduced to 1½ cups, 20 to 25 minutes. Stir in the cashew milk and vegan butter, and heat over low until the butter melts.

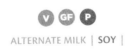

ALTERNATE MILK | **SOY** |

MISO-GINGER DRESSING

Drizzle this gingery dressing over avocados, tomatoes, and shredded cabbage. You could also try it as a sauce for tofu or fish. • **MAKES ½ CUP**

½ teaspoon sliced fresh ginger
½ teaspoon sliced garlic
½ teaspoon sliced jalapeño
3 tablespoons safflower oil
3 tablespoons plain unsweetened coconut
  milk beverage (not canned)

2 tablespoons red miso
2 tablespoons fresh, strained lime juice
1 teaspoon agave nectar

ADD the first three ingredients to the bowl of a mini food processor, and process until finely chopped, about 10 seconds. Add the remaining ingredients, and process until smooth, about 50 seconds.

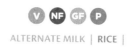

ALTERNATE MILK | RICE |

MANGO-LIME DRESSING

Toss this low-fat tropical dressing with chickpeas and diced tomato and red onion. Or, drizzle over fish. If you use frozen mango, thaw first. ● **MAKES ¾ CUP**

1 teaspoon sliced fresh ginger
½ teaspoon sliced garlic
½ cup diced mango
3 tablespoons plain unsweetened rice milk

3 tablespoons safflower oil
3 tablespoons fresh, strained lime juice
2 teaspoons agave nectar
¼ teaspoon kosher salt

ADD the first two ingredients to the bowl of a mini food processor, and process until finely chopped, about 10 seconds. Add the remaining ingredients, and process until smooth, about 50 seconds.

ALTERNATE MILK | COCONUT | CASHEW |

BREADS & SWEETS

COCONUT

BANOFFEE PIE

"BUTTERMILK" CORNBREAD
WITH BROWN SUGAR

BANANA CHOCOLATE CHIP
MUFFINS

STRAWBERRY "BUTTERMILK"
SHERBET

VEGAN CHOCOLATE–
CHOCOLATE CHIP ICE CREAM
WITH ESPRESSO

FIVE-INGREDIENT VEGAN
VANILLA ICE CREAM

CHERRIES IN CREAM

PALEO PEANUT BUTTER–
CHOCOLATE CHIP COOKIES

COCONUT STICKY RICE WITH
MANGO, LIME, AND HONEY

MATCHA PEACH ICE POPS

CHERRY-LIME ICE POPS

INDIAN PUDDING MUFFINS

CASHEW

DARK CHOCOLATE TRUFFLES
WITH CINNAMON AND CAYENNE

STRAWBERRY CORNBREAD
WITH COCONUT SUGAR

TRIPLE CHOCOLATE
CUPCAKES

FUDGY FLOURLESS
BROWNIES

STRAWBERRY SHORTCAKE
WITH FRESH LEMON ZEST

SOY

WHOLE-WHEAT CHALLAH
WITH RAISINS

DIETARY CATEGORIES: VEGAN VEGETARIAN NUT-FREE GLUTEN-FREE **P** PALEO

GINGERBREAD WITH PRUNES
AND COCOA

ALMOND

VEGAN BLUEBERRY CREAM
TART

SPICED CHOCOLATE MOUSSE
WITH FRESH RASPBERRIES

MATCHA VANILLA MUFFINS

RICE

ROSEMARY POPOVERS

OAT

TRIPLE SEED CAKE WITH
LEMON AND VANILLA

PISTACHIO

STRAWBERRIES WITH
PISTACHIO CREAM

HEMP

DARK CHOCOLATE CHERRY
SCONES

QUINOA

CRANBERRY-WALNUT QUICK
BREAD

HAZELNUT

APPLE COBBLER WITH
GOLDEN RAISINS AND NUTS

FIG AND HAZELNUT
CLAFOUTI WITH ALMOND
AND ORANGE

PUDDINGS

CARDAMOM PUDDING

VANILLA WALNUT PUDDING

HAZELNUT CINNAMON
PUDDING

CURRIED CASHEW PUDDING

COFFEE ALMOND PUDDING

KEY LIME "CHEESECAKE"
MOUSSE

GRAHAM CRACKER PUDDING

GREEN TEA–GINGER PUDDING

MEXICAN CHOCOLATE
PUDDING

LEMON TAPIOCA PUDDING

TOPPINGS

VANILLA ALMOND CREAM

BASIC SWEET GLAZE

SWEET CREAMY ICING

WHIPPED COCONUT CREAM

BANOFFEE PIE

British dessert banoffee pie, or banana-toffee pie, was the inspiration for this dessert. For the best texture, let chill for a few hours. If you don't have graham cracker crumbs, make your own by transferring graham crackers to a bag. Seal the bag and bang with a rolling pin, the bottom of a pot, or the smooth side of a meat mallet. • **SERVES 8**

FOR THE CRUST

2 cups graham cracker crumbs
  (about 11 graham crackers)

1 tablespoon coconut sugar

3 tablespoons mashed ripe banana
  (about ½ small banana)

3 tablespoons vegan butter, melted

¼ teaspoon kosher salt

FOR THE FILLING

3 cups canned (full-fat) coconut milk
  (almost two 15-ounce cans), well shaken

½ cup shredded unsweetened coconut

½ cup coconut sugar

3 tablespoons cornstarch

¼ teaspoon plus ⅛ teaspoon kosher salt

3 large egg yolks (not whole eggs)

2 tablespoons vegan butter

2 teaspoons vanilla extract

About 3 large ripe, but still firm, bananas

¼ cup coconut flakes, lightly toasted, or
  ¼ cup shaved semisweet chocolate

MAKE THE CRUST: Preheat the oven to 350 degrees F, and place a rack in the center. In a medium bowl, stir together the crust ingredients until well blended, and press into the bottom and sides of a 9-inch glass pie dish (the crust won't come all the way up the sides). Chill for 30 minutes, and bake until light golden brown, about 15 minutes. Cool completely at room temperature.

MEANWHILE, MAKE THE FILLING: Heat the coconut milk and shredded coconut in a medium saucepan on medium heat until warm (do not let a skin form). In a medium-large saucepan, whisk together the sugar, cornstarch, and salt. Pour

in the warm milk-coconut mixture, whisking. Cook over medium heat, whisking constantly, until slightly thickened, 2 to 3 minutes. Add the eggs to a small-medium bowl, and whisk until smooth. Stir about ¼ cup of the hot milk-sugar mixture into the eggs, whisking constantly. Pour the egg–hot milk mixture back into the pot with the milk and sugar. Cook, whisking frequently, until the custard comes to a boil and thickens, 3 to 4 minutes. Remove from the heat, and whisk in the vegan butter and vanilla. Let cool to room temperature, then cover with a piece of plastic wrap, and chill until cold, about 1 hour.

SLICE the bananas ¼ inch thick (you need about 2 cups), and arrange in the cooled pie shell. Stir the custard to loosen, and pour over the bananas (the custard should come to about the top of the pie dish). Top evenly with the coconut flakes. Chill until the filling has set, at least 4 hours or overnight.

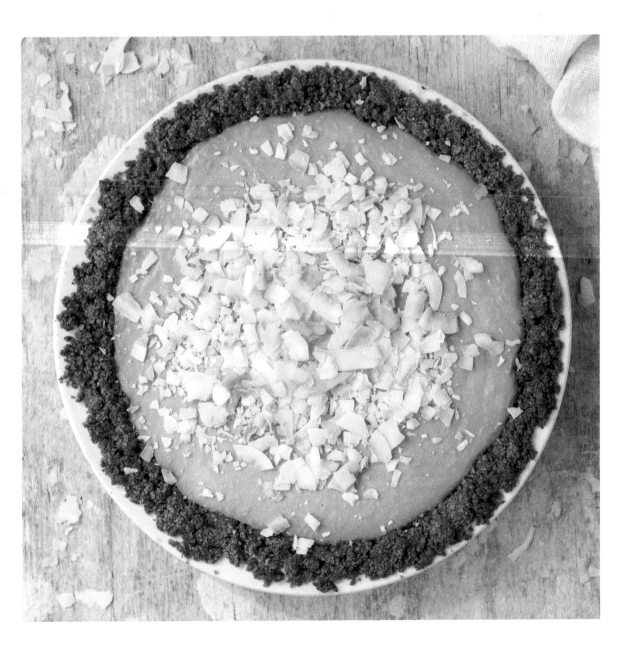

"BUTTERMILK" CORNBREAD WITH BROWN SUGAR

Try pairing this moist cornbread with sliced peaches and vegan vanilla ice cream. Medium-grind cornmeal makes for a more textured, rustic cornbread, but you can go with finely ground. For a vegan version, replace the eggs with two tablespoons of ground flaxseeds mixed with water. • **MAKES 9 SLICES**

Cooking spray

1 cup plus 2 tablespoons plain unsweetened coconut milk beverage (not canned), well shaken

1 tablespoon fresh, strained lemon juice

½ cup (4 tablespoons) vegan butter, melted (and still warm)

½ cup Sucanat or brown sugar

2 large eggs

1 teaspoon vanilla extract

1 cup medium-grind cornmeal

1 cup white whole-wheat flour

½ teaspoon kosher salt

½ teaspoon baking soda

PREHEAT the oven to 375 degrees F. Spray the inside of an 8 x 8-inch baking dish with cooking spray. In a large bowl, whisk together coconut milk and lemon juice, and let sit at room temperature for at least 5 minutes. Then, whisk in the melted vegan butter, Sucanat, eggs, and vanilla.

IN a medium bowl, whisk together the cornmeal, flour, salt, and baking soda. Add to the wet mixture, and whisk just until combined.

POUR into the baking dish, and bake until a tester inserted into the center comes out with only a few crumbs, about 30 minutes. Let cool for 10 minutes, and cut into 9 slices.

ALTERNATE MILK | CASHEW | SOY |

BANANA CHOCOLATE CHIP MUFFINS

These muffins are most delicious warm, when the chocolate chips are still molten (unless they're milk chocolate, they should be dairy-free). Whole-wheat pastry flour makes them very light and airy; however, you can use all white whole-wheat flour. As bananas ripen, transfer them to the fridge and keep them there until they're very dark. • **MAKES 12**

1 cup whole-wheat pastry flour

1 cup plus 1 tablespoon white whole-wheat flour, divided

¼ cup Sucanat or brown sugar

1½ teaspoons baking powder

¾ teaspoon coarse kosher salt

½ teaspoon baking soda

1 heaping packed cup mashed very ripe banana (about 3 small)

1 cup plain unsweetened coconut milk beverage

¼ cup safflower oil

2 large eggs

2 teaspoons vanilla extract

¾ cup semisweet or bittersweet chocolate chips

Nonstick cooking spray

PREHEAT the oven to 375 degrees F. In a large bowl, whisk together all of the whole-wheat pastry flour, 1 cup of the white whole-wheat flour, the Sucanat, baking powder, salt, and baking soda until well blended.

IN a medium bowl, stir together the banana with the coconut milk, oil, eggs, and vanilla, and mash with a potato masher until smooth. Pour the wet mix into the dry mix, and stir just until combined.

MEANWHILE, in a small bowl, toss the chocolate chips with the remaining tablespoon of flour until evenly coated. Pour into the batter and stir just until evenly distributed.

SPRAY the wells of a standard 12-cup muffin pan with cooking spray. Using an ice scream scoop, dollop the batter evenly among the wells. Bake until a tester inserted into the center of a muffin comes out with just a few crumbs, about 20 minutes.

ALTERNATE MILK | RICE | CASHEW |

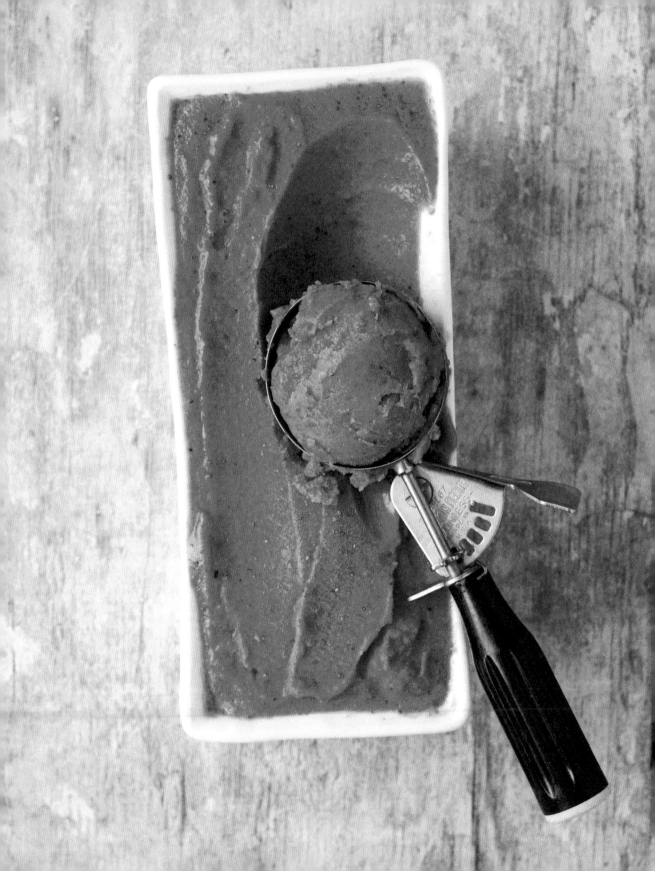

STRAWBERRY "BUTTERMILK" SHERBET

Sherbet is similar to sorbet, but contains a small amount of milk. Red wine vinegar might sound unorthodox, but it melds with coconut milk to form a vegan buttermilk, which adds tanginess to this deep-red sherbet. ● **MAKES 3 CUPS (ABOUT 3 SERVINGS)**

1 cup plain unsweetened coconut milk beverage (not canned)

1 tablespoon red wine vinegar

3 cups hulled strawberries (about 22 ounces)

¾ cup agave nectar

1 teaspoon vanilla extract

¼ teaspoon kosher salt

IN a small bowl, stir together coconut milk and vinegar, and let sit for 10 minutes. Pour into the food processor, and add the remaining ingredients. Puree until very smooth, about 1 minute. Chill, covered, until very cold, at least 2 hours.

FREEZE in an ice cream maker, following the manufacturer's instructions (the churning process should take about 20 minutes). Scoop into a container, and freeze until the sherbet solidifies further, at least 3 hours.

ALTERNATE MILK | CASHEW | CANNED LOW-FAT COCONUT |

VEGAN CHOCOLATE– CHOCOLATE CHIP ICE CREAM WITH ESPRESSO

For chocolate ice cream, omit the espresso powder and—if desired—the chocolate chips. Make sure to use coconut oil, rather than coconut butter, and to use small chocolate chips or small pieces of chopped bar chocolate. Place the ice cream maker insert in the freezer twenty-four hours before preparing this recipe. When you're ready to serve, set the ice cream out for fifteen minutes at room temperature to soften. • **MAKES ABOUT 3 CUPS**

2½ cups canned full-fat coconut milk (about 1½ 13.5-ounce cans), well shaken
½ cup plus 3 tablespoons granulated sugar
⅓ cup unsweetened cocoa powder
¼ cup plus 1 tablespoon coconut oil
2 teaspoons espresso powder

1 teaspoon pure vanilla extract
⅛ teaspoon kosher salt
½ cup dark or semisweet (dairy-free) chocolate chips or small pieces of chopped chocolate

IN a blender, puree all of the ingredients except the chocolate chips until smooth, about 1 minute. Pour into a container, cover, and chill until very cold, several hours or, ideally, overnight.

REMOVE the mixture from the fridge and stir very well until it resembles a smooth custard.

SCRAPE into an ice cream maker, and churn, following the machine's instructions. Once the ice cream reaches soft-serve consistency, add the chocolate chips and churn for another couple of minutes to mix well. Pour into a container, smooth the top, and freeze until hardened, at least 3 hours.

FIVE-INGREDIENT VEGAN VANILLA ICE CREAM

I highly recommend Nielsen-Massey vanilla bean paste (available at Whole Foods Markets and many gourmet grocers or online) or the seeds from a vanilla bean for this easy-to-prepare vegan ice cream. Not only will it give the treat a super-intense vanilla flavor—it will also impart small brown flecks revealing the presence of real vanilla bean. However, two teaspoons of pure vanilla extract will do in a pinch. Make sure to use coconut oil, rather than coconut butter, and to place the ice cream maker insert in the freezer twenty-four hours before preparing this recipe. When you're ready to serve, set the ice cream out for fifteen minutes at room temperature to soften. • **MAKES ABOUT 2½ CUPS**

2½ cups canned full-fat coconut milk (about 1½ 13.5-ounce cans), well shaken

½ cup granulated sugar

¼ cup plus 1 tablespoon coconut oil

2 teaspoons vanilla bean paste or the seeds from a vanilla bean

⅛ teaspoon kosher salt

IN a blender, puree all of the ingredients until smooth, about 1 minute. Pour into a container, cover, and chill until very cold, several hours or, ideally, overnight.

REMOVE the mixture from the fridge and stir very well until it resembles a smooth custard.

SCRAPE the mixture into an ice cream maker, and churn, following the machine's instructions. Pour into a container, smooth the top, and freeze until hardened, at least 3 hours.

CHERRIES IN CREAM

Try this recipe with different fruit, such as strawberries, peaches, mangoes, or pineapples. You can find coconut cream (not full-fat coconut milk or the sweetened coconut cream product meant for cocktails) at Trader Joe's, Whole Foods, and natural food stores. • **SERVES 4**

4 cups pitted fresh sweet cherries
¼ cup strained fresh orange juice
3 tablespoons agave nectar, divided
1 teaspoon vanilla extract

¼ teaspoon kosher salt
1 cup canned coconut cream (from a well-shaken can)

IN a medium bowl, stir together the cherries, orange juice, 2 tablespoons of the agave nectar, the vanilla, and the salt. Let sit for at least 15 minutes at room temperature. In a small bowl, stir together the remaining agave nectar plus the coconut cream.

LADLE the cherries and their juices into 4 small bowls, and top with the coconut cream.

PALEO PEANUT BUTTER– CHOCOLATE CHIP COOKIES

Low-sugar and rich in fiber and protein, these easy-to-prepare cookies are delicious and guilt-free! Serve with a glass of cold coconut milk to reinforce the coconut flavor. • **MAKES 13**

1½ cups tiger nut flour, such as Organic Gemini
½ cup finely shredded unsweetened coconut
1 teaspoon baking powder
¼ teaspoon salt
¼ cup plus 2 tablespoons unsweetened coconut milk beverage (or canned coconut milk)

¼ cup creamy peanut butter (with salt, without sugar)
¼ cup agave nectar
2 teaspoons pure vanilla extract
⅓ cup semisweet or dark chocolate chips

PREHEAT the oven to 375 degrees F, place a rack in the center of the oven, and line a baking sheet with parchment paper. In a large bowl, stir together the tiger nut flour, coconut, baking powder, and salt. Add the coconut milk, peanut butter, agave nectar, and vanilla extract, and stir until well mixed. Stir in the chocolate chips until evenly distributed.

USING an ice cream scoop, scoop rounds onto the parchment, spacing them about 1 inch apart. Flatten each round a bit with your palm. Bake until the cookies are golden brown, about 15 minutes.

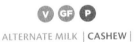

ALTERNATE MILK | **CASHEW** |

COCONUT STICKY RICE WITH MANGO, LIME, AND HONEY

Ripe mangoes inspired my take on the classic Thai dessert: coconut sticky rice with mango. This 6-ingredient recipe is simple to prepare, and delicious as a breakfast, dessert, or snack. ● **MAKES 4 SERVINGS**

2 cups plain unsweetened coconut milk, refrigerated beverage or canned

2 cups water

Zest of 2 small limes, all white pith removed, minced, divided

½ teaspoon salt

1 cup sushi rice (white)

2 tablespoons agave nectar, plus another teaspoon for drizzling

2 ripe mangoes, sliced

ADD coconut milk, 2 cups water, three quarters of the zest, and the salt to a medium saucepot, and bring to a boil over high heat. Immediately stir in the rice. Cover and simmer over low heat for 15 minutes. Remove from the heat and let sit, covered, for another 10 minutes. Stir in 2 table-spoons of the honey. Ladle into 4 small-medium serving bowls.

TOP each serving with mango slices, sprinkle with the remaining minced lime zest, and drizzle evenly with the remaining teaspoon of honey. Serve.

MATCHA PEACH ICE POPS

Matcha green tea powder flavors and colors these refreshing ice pops. ● **MAKES 10**

2¾ cups unsweetened frozen peaches
   (1 10-ounce bag)
1¾ cups plain unsweetened coconut milk
   beverage

¼ cup agave nectar
¼ teaspoon salt
2 teaspoons matcha powder

ADD the first four ingredients to a blender. In a small bowl, whisk together 1 tablespoon very hot water and the matcha until well mixed, and scrape into the blender. Puree until smooth, about 1 minute.

POUR into a 10-pop ice pop mold, cover, and freeze until firm, at least 2 hours.

CHERRY-LIME ICE POPS

Frozen cherries are so sweet: only a hint of agave nectar is needed. You've been warned: these pops are messy, so serve outside, letting them drip freely onto your patio or deck! • **MAKES 9.**

2 cups frozen sweet cherries
1 cup plain unsweetened coconut milk
  beverage

¼ cup agave nectar
1 tablespoon fresh, strained lime juice
⅛ teaspoon salt

IN a blender, puree all of the ingredients until smooth, about 1 minute. Pour into an ice pop mold, and freeze until solid, at least 2 hours. Place the bottom of the mold in a bowl of warm water for a minute or so to make releasing the pops easier.

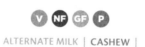

ALTERNATE MILK | CASHEW |

INDIAN PUDDING MUFFINS

Use up leftover ripe bananas in these delicious muffins, inspired by the traditional American dessert. • **MAKES 12**

Cooking spray
2 medium very ripe bananas, mashed
1 cup plain unsweetened coconut milk
(canned or refrigerated beverage)
2 large eggs
½ cup molasses

1 cup fine ground cornmeal
1 cup white whole-wheat flour
¼ cup granulated sugar
2 teaspoons baking powder
½ teaspoon baking soda
½ teaspoon salt

PREHEAT the oven to 350 degrees F, and spray a 12-well muffin pan with cooking spray. In a large bowl, stir together mashed banana, coconut milk, eggs, and molasses. In a medium bowl, whisk together cornmeal, flour, sugar, baking powder, baking soda, and salt. Pour the dry ingredients into the wet ingredients, and stir together.

USING a ¼-cup measure, dollop the batter among the wells in the muffin pan. Bake until only a couple of crumbs cling to a cake tester when inserted into the center of a muffin, about 25 minutes.

LET cool in the pan for 15 minutes, then transfer to a cooling rack.

ALTERNATE MILK | CASHEW |

DARK CHOCOLATE TRUFFLES WITH CINNAMON AND CAYENNE

These spiced truffles really do resemble the luxe mushrooms. For ease in shaping, let the chilled chocolate mixture sit at room temperature for about 10 minutes beforehand.

● **MAKES SEVEN 1-INCH TRUFFLES**

3½ ounces 70%-cacao high-quality dark
   chocolate, chopped
¼ cup plain unsweetened cashew milk
2 tablespoons vegan butter
¼ teaspoon ground cinnamon

¼ teaspoon kosher salt
⅛ teaspoon cayenne pepper
3 tablespoons coconut sugar
2 teaspoons unsweetened cocoa powder

PLACE the chocolate in a medium microwave-safe bowl. Microwave in 20-second increments at high power, stirring after each, until 90 percent melted, about 2 minutes. Whisk until smooth.

WHISK in the cashew milk, vegan butter, cinnamon, salt, and cayenne until smooth. Cover and chill until hardened and cold, at least 1 hour.

MIX the coconut sugar and cocoa powder in a small-medium bowl.

USE a spoon and your hands to form 1-inch-diameter balls of the chocolate mixture. Add one at a time to the sugar mixture. Roll around to coat, making the balls more round. When finished rolling all of the truffles, cover, and chill until firm, about 1 hour. Serve either slightly chilled or at room temperature.

ALTERNATE MILK | COCONUT | SOY |

STRAWBERRY CORNBREAD WITH COCONUT SUGAR

This tender, lightly sweetened whole-grain quick bread is simple to prepare and wholesome. To make it more decadent, drizzle with pure maple syrup before serving. • **SERVES 8**

Nonstick cooking spray

1 cup corn flour or fine-ground cornmeal

1 cup white whole-wheat flour or
  whole-wheat flour

¼ cup coconut sugar, brown sugar, or Sucanat

2 teaspoons baking powder

½ teaspoon salt

¼ teaspoon baking soda

1½ cups unsweetened cashew milk

¼ cup safflower or olive oil

2 large eggs

2 teaspoons vanilla extract

1 cup halved, hulled small strawberries,
  preferably local

SPRAY an 8 x 8-inch baking dish with cooking spray, and preheat the oven to 350 degrees F.

IN a medium bowl, whisk together cornmeal, flour, sugar, baking powder, salt, and baking soda. In a large bowl, whisk together cashew milk, oil, eggs, and vanilla.

POUR the batter into the greased baking dish. Arrange the strawberry halves around the top. Bake until a tester inserted into the center comes out with just a couple of crumbs, about 35 minutes.

ALTERNATE MILK | COCONUT | SOY |

TRIPLE CHOCOLATE CUPCAKES

These chocolate–chocolate chip cupcakes are topped with a vegan chocolate glaze, for an elegant, decadent dessert. Frosting them while still warm makes for moister cupcakes and a more rustic look; doing so while at room temperature results in a more elegant appearance. • **MAKES 12**

½ cup plus 2 tablespoons all-purpose flour
½ cup plus 2 tablespoons plus 1 teaspoon
   whole-wheat pastry flour, divided
¼ cup unsweetened cocoa powder
1 teaspoon baking powder
½ teaspoon baking soda
½ teaspoon kosher salt
2 large eggs

½ cup coconut sugar
½ cup safflower oil
1 tablespoon pure vanilla extract, divided
¾ cup plain unsweetened cashew milk,
   divided
¾ cup semisweet chocolate chips, divided
2 tablespoons vegan butter

PREHEAT the oven to 350 degrees F, and place a rack in the center. Place paper cupcake liners in the wells of a standard 12-cup cupcake or muffin pan. In a medium bowl, whisk together all of the all-purpose flour, ½ cup plus 2 tablespoons of the whole-wheat pastry flour, the cocoa powder, baking powder, baking soda, and salt until well mixed.

ADD the eggs to the bowl of an electric mixer (fitted with the paddle attachment), and beat on medium until smooth, about 20 seconds. Add the sugar, and beat until incorporated well, about 30 seconds. Add the oil and 2 teaspoons of the vanilla, and beat until the mixture is relatively smooth, about another minute.

REDUCE the speed to medium low. Add half of the flour mixture and beat for 10 seconds. Add 6 tablespoons of the milk and beat for 10 sec-

onds. Add the remaining flour mixture and beat for 10 seconds. Add another 5 tablespoons of the milk (1 tablespoon of milk should remain) and beat for 10 seconds. With a rubber spatula, scrape down the sides of the bowl to incorporate and beat just until smooth and well mixed, about another 10 seconds (do not overmix).

TO a small bowl, add ¼ cup of the chocolate chips plus the remaining teaspoon of whole-wheat pastry flour, and toss together. Pour the mixture into the batter and mix on low just until incorporated, about 5 seconds.

POUR the batter into the cupcake liners (you will add about ¼ cup to each), and bake until a tester inserted into the center comes out with only a few crumbs, 17 to 20 minutes. Let cool in the pan for 5 minutes, then carefully transfer to a cooling rack.

MEANWHILE, add the remaining tablespoon of cashew milk plus the remaining ½ cup chocolate chips and the vegan butter to a medium, microwave-safe bowl. Microwave at high power for 40 seconds. Add the remaining teaspoon of vanilla extract, and stir until the chocolate has all melted and the mixture is smooth (you should have ⅓ cup).

WHILE the cupcakes are still warm, evenly spread the glaze over their tops with a small offset spatula or the back of a spoon.

ALTERNATE MILK | SOY | COCONUT | HAZELNUT |

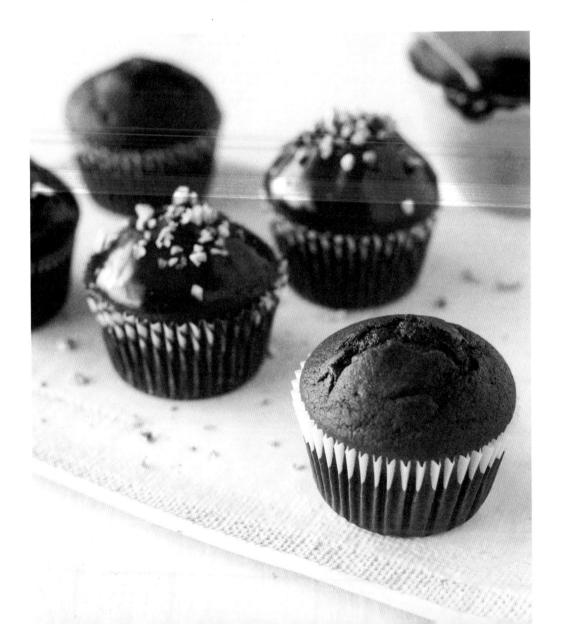

FUDGY FLOURLESS BROWNIES

Cashew flour and milk lend these rich brownies a moist, almost fudgy texture. Dark or semisweet chocolate (rather than milk or white) should be dairy-free; however, check the label to be sure. Don't forget to sift the nut flour or meal well to remove any lumps. And for a neat presentation, it's important to chill the brownies until very cold before slicing. Serve with fresh berries and Whipped Coconut Cream (page 121). • **MAKES 8 MEDIUM OR 16 SMALL BROWNIES (ABOUT 8 SERVINGS)**

Nonstick cooking spray

1 cup cashew or almond flour or meal, well sifted

¼ cup unsweetened cocoa powder

¾ cup plus 2 tablespoons coconut sugar or brown sugar

¼ cup granulated sugar

2 teaspoons baking powder

¼ teaspoon baking soda

¼ teaspoon kosher salt

1 stick (8 tablespoons) vegan butter, melted

2 ounces (dairy-free) semisweet or dark chocolate (such as 60% cacao) in bar form, melted

2 large eggs, lightly beaten

¼ cup plain unsweetened cashew milk

2 tablespoons safflower oil

1 teaspoon vanilla extract

PREHEAT the oven to 350 degrees F, and grease an 8 x 8-inch baking dish with cooking spray.

IN a medium bowl, whisk together the cashew flour, cocoa powder, coconut sugar, granulated sugar, baking powder, baking soda, and salt.

IN a large bowl, stir together the melted vegan butter and melted chocolate. Allow to cool slightly until warm, not hot. Whisk in the eggs, cashew milk, oil, and vanilla. Pour the dry mixture into this wet mixture, and stir just until combined (do not overmix).

POUR the batter into the greased baking dish. Bake on the center rack until a tester poked into the center comes out with just a few moist crumbs, about 25 minutes. (The sides of the brownies will pull away from the perimeter of the pan and the center will sink slightly—this is normal.) Let cool to room temperature, at least 30 minutes.

COVER and chill until very cold, at least 2 hours. Cut into squares. (If you try to cut into the brownies before they're cold, they won't form neat squares or rectangles.)

ALTERNATE MILK | HAZELNUT | ALMOND |

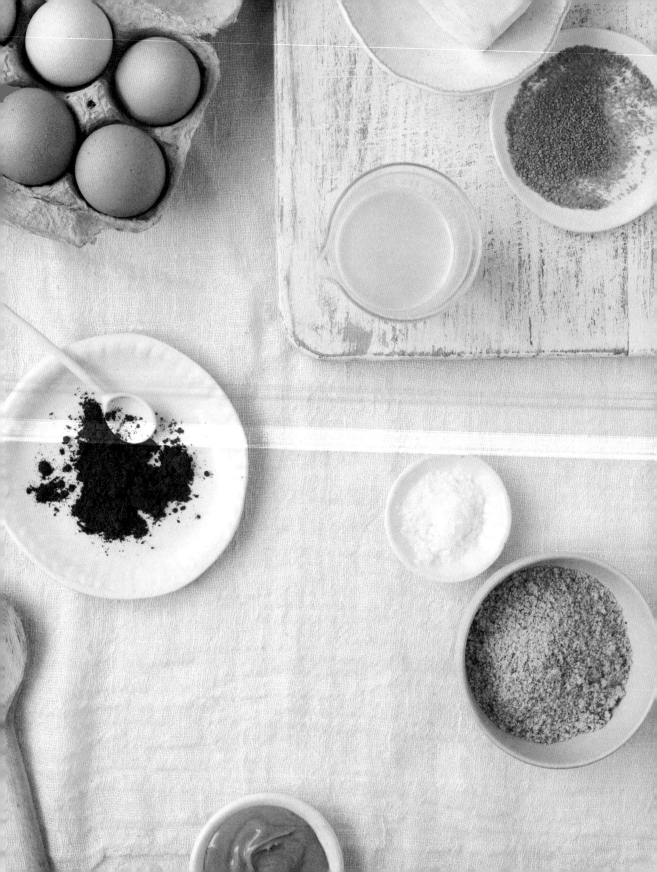

STRAWBERRY SHORTCAKE WITH FRESH LEMON ZEST

Try varying the recipe with mango, pineapple, and kiwi or another type of berry instead of the strawberries. The sweet, fluffy, thick biscuits are also incredibly delicious on their own, split and served with preserves. • **SERVES 8**

FOR THE BISCUITS
About 3 cups all-purpose flour, divided
3 tablespoons granulated sugar
1 tablespoon baking powder
½ teaspoon kosher salt
7 tablespoons vegan butter (very cold)
1 cup plus 2 tablespoons plain unsweetened
   cashew milk (very cold), divided
1½ teaspoons vanilla extract

FOR THE FILLING
2 pounds strawberries, hulled and sliced
   (about 8 cups)
3 tablespoons granulated sugar
1 tablespoon freshly grated lemon zest
   (about 2 large lemons)

FOR ASSEMBLY
1½ cups Whipped Coconut Cream (page 121)
   or 8 scoops (1 recipe) Five-Ingredient
   Vegan Vanilla Ice Cream (page 75)

FOR THE BISCUITS: Preheat the oven to 450 degrees F and place a rack in the upper third of the oven. Line a baking sheet with parchment paper.

IN a medium-large bowl, whisk together 2½ cups of the flour with the sugar, baking powder, and salt until well blended. Cut the butter into small cubes, and add to the flour mixture. Use your fingers to crumble the butter into the dry mixture, until the dough attains the texture of coarse meal (you still want there to be lots of butter bits, for flakiness).

IN a small-medium bowl, whisk together 1 cup of the cashew milk plus the vanilla. Pour it into the dry mix, and gently knead just until a smooth dough forms (if it's still very sticky, begin adding the remaining flour 2 tablespoons at a time, up to a total of 3 cups maximum, but avoid overworking the dough).

POUR the dough onto a cold clean surface, and pat down into a roughly 4 x 4-inch rectangle 1 inch thick. With a sharp biscuit cutter (ideally with a 2-inch diameter), cut into about 8 rounds. Transfer to the lined baking sheet, spacing them at least 1 inch from each other.

BRUSH the remaining 2 tablespoons cashew milk on top of the biscuits. Immediately transfer to the oven, and bake until slightly golden brown on the bottom and cooked through, about 12 minutes. Split each one in half (if saving for another use, keep whole).

FOR THE FILLING: While the biscuits bake, stir together the strawberries, sugar, and lemon zest in a large bowl, until well combined. (This can be done up to 1 hour in advance.)

TO ASSEMBLE: On each of 8 serving plates, place a warm split biscuit. Spoon berry mixture and then whipped cream or ice cream on top. Serve.

ALTERNATE MILK | SOY | COCONUT |

WHOLE-WHEAT CHALLAH WITH RAISINS

Challah, a Jewish Sabbath bread, is puffy, tender, and sweet. Best served warm, it's over-the-top delicious dipped into honey. Microwaving the milk for forty to fifty seconds should bring it to the right temperature—it should feel warm, but not hot.

● **MAKES 1 LARGE LOAF**

¾ cup plain unsweetened soy milk, heated to about 115 degrees F

1 teaspoon coconut sugar

1 packet active dry yeast (about 2 teaspoons)

2 cups white whole-wheat flour

2 cups plus 1 tablespoon all-purpose flour, divided

1¼ teaspoons kosher salt

½ cup plus 1 tablespoon olive oil, divided

½ cup honey

2 large eggs plus 1 large egg yolk, divided

⅓ cup raisins

POUR the warmed soy milk into a large bowl, and whisk in the sugar and yeast. Stir and let sit until foamy, about 10 minutes. Meanwhile, in a medium-large bowl, whisk together the whole-wheat flour, 2 cups of the all-purpose flour, and the salt.

TO the milk-sugar-yeast mixture, add ½ cup of the oil, the honey, and 2 of the eggs, and whisk until blended. Add the flour-salt mix, and stir until blended. Add the raisins, and stir until incorporated.

SPRINKLE the remaining tablespoon of flour onto a large, clean surface. Place the dough ball

on top, and knead until smooth, about 5 minutes (if very sticky, incorporate that flour into the dough).

BRUSH the inside of a medium-large bowl with the remaining tablespoon of oil. Add the dough, cover, and let sit in a warm place until doubled in size, about 1 hour. Punch down, re-cover, and let sit until puffed up, about 30 minutes.

WITH a knife or bench scraper, divide the dough into 3 equal pieces. Line a baking sheet with parchment paper, and transfer the dough pieces onto the parchment. Shape each one into a 16-inch-long rope. Arrange the ropes side-by-side perpendicular to you. Pinch the ends of the strands together to form one end of the loaf (at the ends farthest from you). Weave the three strands together to form a braid. Cover and let sit until doubled, about 1 hour 15 minutes.

PREHEAT the oven to 350 degrees F, and place a rack in the center. In a small bowl, whisk together the egg yolk with 1 tablespoon water until smooth. Brush the challah with some of the egg wash. Bake until golden brown and cooked through in the center, about 35 minutes.

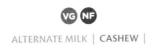

ALTERNATE MILK | CASHEW |

GINGERBREAD WITH PRUNES AND COCOA

Cocoa powder and prunes are the secret ingredients in this ultra-moist gingerbread. Prune puree keeps the fat content down, while adding flavor. Try serving plain, with vegan butter (mixed with fresh orange zest and agave nectar), or with vegan ice cream.

● **MAKES 8 LARGE SLICES**

Nonstick cooking spray

½ cup plain unsweetened soy milk, well shaken

1 tablespoon fresh, strained lemon juice

1 heaping teaspoon freshly grated ginger (about 1-inch piece)

½ cup pitted prunes (about 14)

5 tablespoons boiling water

1½ cups white whole-wheat flour

1 tablespoon unsweetened cocoa powder

1 teaspoon ground cinnamon

½ teaspoon baking soda

½ teaspoon kosher salt

½ teaspoon ground allspice

½ teaspoon ground cloves

5 tablespoons vegan butter, at room temperature

½ cup Sucanat or brown sugar

½ cup molasses (unsulfured)

2 large eggs

PREHEAT the oven to 350 degrees F, and position a rack in the center of the oven. Spray the inside of an 8 x 8-inch baking dish with cooking spray. Measure the soy milk into a liquid measuring cup, and stir in the lemon juice. Let sit at room temperature for 10 to 15 minutes. Stir in the ginger.

MEANWHILE, in a mini food processor, puree the prunes with the boiling water until smooth, about 40 seconds (you should have ½ cup puree).

IN a large bowl, whisk together the flour, cocoa, cinnamon, baking soda, salt, allspice, and cloves until no clumps remain.

IN the bowl of a standing mixer, mix the vegan butter and Sucanat on medium-high speed until fluffy and lighter in color, 4 to 5 minutes. Add the molasses, and blend until well mixed, about 30 seconds. Add the prune puree and eggs and mix until well blended, about 30 seconds.

ADD one third of the flour mixture, and mix on low speed just until blended, about 10 seconds. Add half of the soy milk mixture and mix on low speed just until blended, about 10 seconds. Add another third of the flour mixture and mix on low just until blended, 10 seconds. Add the remaining soy milk mixture and mix on low just until blended, 10 seconds. Add the remaining flour mixture and mix on low just until blended, 10 seconds. (During this process, use a spatula to scrape down the sides of the bowl to make sure everything in the batter mixture is incorporated.)

POUR the batter into the greased baking dish, and bake until a tester poked into the center comes out with just a few crumbs, about 40 minutes.

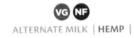

ALTERNATE MILK | HEMP |

VEGAN BLUEBERRY CREAM TART

In this vegan tart, silky vanilla custard meets fresh blueberries and a whole-grain graham cracker–like crust. For an even quicker dessert, use a store-bought pie shell. • **SERVES 8**

1½ cups plus 3 tablespoons white whole-wheat flour, divided
¼ cup Sucanat or brown sugar
1 teaspoon coarse kosher salt, divided
½ teaspoon ground cinnamon
1 stick (8 tablespoons) plus 3 tablespoons vegan butter, chilled and cubed
5 tablespoons plain unsweetened almond milk, divided

1 tablespoon flaxseeds, finely ground
3 tablespoons ice-cold water
1½ teaspoons vanilla extract, divided
Nonstick cooking spray
1½ cups plain silken tofu, drained (about 12 ounces)
3 tablespoons agave nectar
1 tablespoon coconut oil
About 1½ cups fresh blueberries

IN a medium bowl, whisk together 1½ cups plus 1 tablespoon of the flour, the Sucanat, ¾ teaspoon of the salt, and the cinnamon until thoroughly mixed. Add the butter, and crumble together until the mixture forms coarse meal.

IN a small bowl, whisk together 3 tablespoons of the almond milk, the flaxseeds, the ice-cold water, and ½ teaspoon of the vanilla. Add to the flour mixture, and massage the dough until it forms a ball. Wrap in plastic and flatten into a 1-inch-thick disk. Chill for at least 30 minutes.

SPRAY the inside of a 9- or 9½-inch round fluted tart pan (with a removable bottom) with cooking spray. Sprinkle the remaining 2 tablespoons of

flour onto a large, clean, cold surface. On this surface, roll out the dough (using a rolling pin and bench scraper) into a circle roughly 12 inches in diameter. After each roll, rotate the dough a quarter turn. Transfer the dough circle to the tart pan. Press it into the bottom and sides, rolling the rolling pin over the surface to remove any excess dough (which you can use for patching holes). Cover with plastic wrap and chill for at least 30 minutes. Meanwhile, preheat the oven to 400 degrees F.

PLACE the tart shell on a baking sheet. Spray a large piece of aluminum foil with cooking spray and place the foil, spray side down, onto the dough in the tart pan. Top with dried beans or pie weights. Bake for 20 minutes. Remove from the oven and take off the foil and weights (discard the foil). Use a fork to poke about 15 holes in the bottom of the shell. Return to the oven and bake until very lightly golden, about another 10 minutes (the crust may shrink a bit). Let cool to room temperature.

TO a mini food processor, add the tofu, agave nectar, remaining 2 tablespoons almond milk, coconut oil, remaining teaspoon of vanilla, and remaining ¼ teaspoon salt. Puree until smooth, about 40 seconds.

RINSE the berries. Spread a clean kitchen towel on the counter, and pour on top, topping with another kitchen towel. Let the berries drain for a few minutes.

POUR and scrape the tofu-agave cream into the crust. Make sure to leave about ⅓ inch of space at the top for the berries (you might have a bit of extra custard). Evenly sprinkle the berries on top. Cover the tart with plastic wrap, and chill in the refrigerator to firm up the custard, at least 2 hours.

ALTERNATE MILK | **COCONUT** |

SPICED CHOCOLATE MOUSSE WITH FRESH RASPBERRIES

This creamy, near-instant pudding is delicious solo. Or, try it in the tart shell of the Vegan Blueberry Cream Tart (page 94) with fresh raspberries instead of blueberries. To melt chocolate, microwave for thirty seconds, stir, and microwave for another twenty seconds or so. Remove from the microwave when the chocolate is 90 percent melted, and stir until smooth. ● **MAKES 1¾ CUPS (ABOUT 4 SMALL SERVINGS)**

1½ cups plain silken tofu, drained (about 12 ounces) and broken up a bit

¼ cup semisweet chocolate chips, melted

3 tablespoons agave nectar

2 tablespoons plain unsweetened almond milk

1 tablespoon coconut oil

2 teaspoons unsweetened cocoa powder

1 teaspoon vanilla extract

¼ teaspoon ground cinnamon

¼ teaspoon kosher salt

About ½ cup fresh raspberries, rinsed and drained

TO a mini food processor, add all of the ingredients except for the berries. Puree until smooth, about 40 seconds. Ladle into 4 small cups, and chill. Before serving, top with the berries.

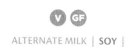

ALTERNATE MILK | **SOY** |

MATCHA VANILLA MUFFINS

To make these green tea treats more decadent, slather with strawberry, matcha, or chocolate frosting. • **MAKES 12**

Cooking spray
1 cup white whole-wheat flour
1 cup all-purpose flour
¾ cup granulated sugar
2 tablespoons matcha powder
2 teaspoons baking powder

½ teaspoon salt
1½ cups plain unsweetened almond milk
¼ cup safflower or vegetable oil
2 large eggs
2 tablespoons vegan butter, melted
2 teaspoons vanilla extract

PREHEAT the oven to 350 degrees F, and spray a standard-size 12-well muffin pan with cooking spray.

IN a medium bowl, whisk together the white whole-wheat flour, all-purpose flour, sugar, matcha, baking powder, and salt. In a large bowl, whisk together the almond milk, oil, eggs, melted vegan butter, and vanilla. Pour the dry into the wet mixture, and stir just until combined (do not overmix).

EVENLY divide the batter among the wells in the greased muffin pan. Bake until only a few crumbs stick to a cake tester when poked into the center of a muffin, about 25 minutes. Let cool in the pan for 10 minutes, then gently transfer muffins to a cooling rack to finish cooling. Serve.

ALTERNATE MILK | COCONUT | CASHEW |

ROSEMARY POPOVERS

Most delicious warm from the oven, these popovers are also puffy and moist at room temperature, paired with pumpkin or apple butter. Instead of brushing them with butter, you can dip them into olive oil. • **MAKES 6**

2 large eggs
1¼ cups plain unsweetened rice milk
½ cup white whole-wheat flour
½ cup all-purpose flour

1 teaspoon minced fresh rosemary leaves
1 teaspoon coconut sugar
½ teaspoon kosher salt
1 tablespoon vegan butter, melted

PREHEAT the oven to 450 degrees F, and place an oven rack in the top third. In a medium bowl, beat the eggs until smooth, about 20 seconds. Add the remaining ingredients (other than the vegan butter), and beat just until smooth.

DIVIDE the batter among the 6 wells of a nonstick popover pan, and place in the hot oven. (If you

don't have a nonstick popover pan, use a regular popover or muffin pan, and grease and flour.)

BAKE for 20 minutes. Reduce the oven temperature to 350 degrees F, and bake until golden brown and puffed on top and cooked through (but still moist) in the center, about another 20 minutes. Brush with vegan butter, and serve immediately.

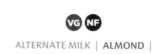

ALTERNATE MILK | **ALMOND** |

TRIPLE SEED CAKE WITH LEMON AND VANILLA

Inspired by lemon poppy seed cake, this golden-brown-on-the-outside, moist-on-the-inside loaf is delicious for breakfast, an afternoon snack, or dessert. Try brushing with a mixture of warm agave nectar and lemon juice after it emerges from the oven. ● **MAKES 1 LOAF**

1½ cups plain unsweetened oat milk
Scant tablespoon fresh, strained lemon juice (about 1 small lemon)
¼ cup light olive oil
¼ cup agave nectar
2 large eggs
1 teaspoon vanilla extract
Zest of 1 lemon (about 1 teaspoon)
1 cup white whole-wheat flour

1 cup whole-wheat pastry flour
¼ cup Sucanat or brown sugar
2 tablespoons white sesame seeds
1 tablespoon chia seeds
1 tablespoon ground flaxseeds
1 teaspoon baking powder
½ teaspoon baking soda
½ teaspoon coarse kosher salt
Nonstick cooking spray

PREHEAT the oven to 375 degrees F, and place a rack in the center.

IN a large bowl, stir together the oat milk and lemon juice, and let sit for 10 minutes. Add the oil, agave nectar, eggs, vanilla, and lemon zest, and whisk well.

IN a medium bowl, whisk together the white whole-wheat flour, whole-wheat pastry flour, Sucanat, sesame seeds, chia seeds, flaxseeds,

baking powder, baking soda, and salt until well combined. Add the dry mix to the wet mix, and stir just until combined (do not overmix).

SPRAY the inside of a roughly 9½ x 4½-inch loaf pan with cooking spray. Pour the batter into the pan. Bake until a fork inserted into the center of the cake comes out with just a few crumbs, about 50 minutes. Let cool for about 10 minutes; turn out onto a flat surface; slice; and serve.

ALTERNATE MILK | RICE | ALMOND |

STRAWBERRIES WITH PISTACHIO CREAM

This nourishing dessert pairs red strawberries with pale green, luscious pistachio cream. It's also delicious with almond, hazelnut, or macadamia nut cream; follow the same recipe, just with different nuts. You can also try fresh blueberries or a mixture of berries on top. Make sure to use raw (not roasted) pistachios for a greener, fresher-tasting cream. • **SERVES 4**

1 cup raw unsalted pistachios
2 tablespoons agave nectar
½ teaspoon almond or vanilla extract
¼ teaspoon kosher salt

1 pint fresh strawberries, hulled and sliced
3 tablespoons finely chopped pistachios
Optional for garnish: 1 teaspoon freshly
    grated orange zest

PLACE the nuts in a medium bowl and cover with a couple of inches of water. Soak for 8 hours.

RINSE and drain the pistachios (they will have increased in volume to about 1½ cups), and transfer to a high-speed blender. Add 1 cup fresh water, the honey, almond extract, and salt, and

puree until smooth, about 1 minute. (You should yield a scant 2 cups pistachio cream.)

SPOON the pistachio cream into 4 small dessert cups or bowls. Arrange the berries on top. Sprinkle with pistachios and, if desired, orange zest. Serve.

ALTERNATE CREAM | ALMOND | PECAN | WALNUT | HAZELNUT | MACADAMIA |

DARK CHOCOLATE CHERRY SCONES

When eaten warm, these brownie-like whole-grain scones feature molten chocolate chips plus a tart cherry kick. Heaven! • **MAKES ABOUT 10**

2 cups plus 1 tablespoon white whole-wheat flour, divided

½ cup plus 1 tablespoon coconut sugar, divided

¼ cup unsweetened cocoa powder

1 tablespoon baking powder

½ teaspoon baking soda

¾ teaspoon kosher salt

6 tablespoons vegan butter, chilled

½ cup plus 1 tablespoon plain unsweetened hemp milk, chilled, divided

2 large eggs

1 teaspoon vanilla extract

½ cup semisweet chocolate chips

⅓ cup sweetened dried cherries

PREHEAT the oven to 375 degrees, and place a rack in the center. Line a baking or cookie sheet with parchment paper.

ADD 2 cups of the white whole-wheat flour; ½ cup of the coconut sugar; and the cocoa powder, baking powder, baking soda, and salt to a medium-large bowl, and whisk until well mixed. Add the vegan butter, and crumble until a coarse meal forms.

IN a large bowl, whisk together ½ cup of the hemp milk, the eggs, and the vanilla until well blended. Add the dry mixture, and stir just until well mixed. Add the chocolate chips and cherries, and mix until distributed evenly.

SPRINKLE the additional tablespoon of white whole-wheat flour onto a clean cold surface. Add the dough, and knead a couple of times until it comes together and becomes smooth (do not overwork). Pat into a ¾- to 1-inch-thick rectangle. Use a round biscuit cutter to cut out about 10 biscuits (form more scones from dough scraps). Transfer to the baking sheet, spacing 1 inch apart.

BRUSH with the remaining tablespoon of hemp milk, and sprinkle with the remaining tablespoon of coconut sugar. Bake until the sugar on top melts and the scones cook through in the center, about 15 minutes.

ALTERNATE MILK | SEVEN-GRAIN | HAZELNUT |

CRANBERRY-WALNUT QUICK BREAD

This cake-like bread is nourishing and incredibly flavorful. If you use plain unsweetened milk,
add a tablespoon or two of extra coconut sugar. • **MAKES 12 BARS**

Nonstick cooking spray
2 cups whole-wheat pastry flour
½ cup coconut sugar
½ teaspoon baking powder
½ teaspoon baking soda
1 teaspoon kosher salt
½ teaspoon ground cinnamon

1¼ cups plain quinoa milk (sweetened)
3 large eggs
4 tablespoons vegan butter, melted and
   cooled to room temperature
1 teaspoon vanilla extract
⅓ cup toasted walnuts, finely chopped
⅓ cup sweetened dried cranberries or cherries

1. PREHEAT the oven to 350 degrees F, and place a rack in the center. Grease a 13 x 9-inch baking dish with cooking spray.

2. IN a medium-large bowl, whisk together the pastry flour, coconut sugar, baking powder, baking soda, salt, and cinnamon until well mixed. In a large bowl, stir together the quinoa milk, eggs, melted vegan butter, and vanilla until well mixed.

Add the dry mixture, and stir just until combined. Stir in the nuts and cranberries.

3. POUR into the baking dish. Bake until a tester inserted into the center comes out with only a few crumbs and the cake is golden brown, about 20 minutes. Let cool to room temperature, and cut into 12 bars.

ALTERNATE MILK | **PLAIN SWEETENED HAZELNUT** |

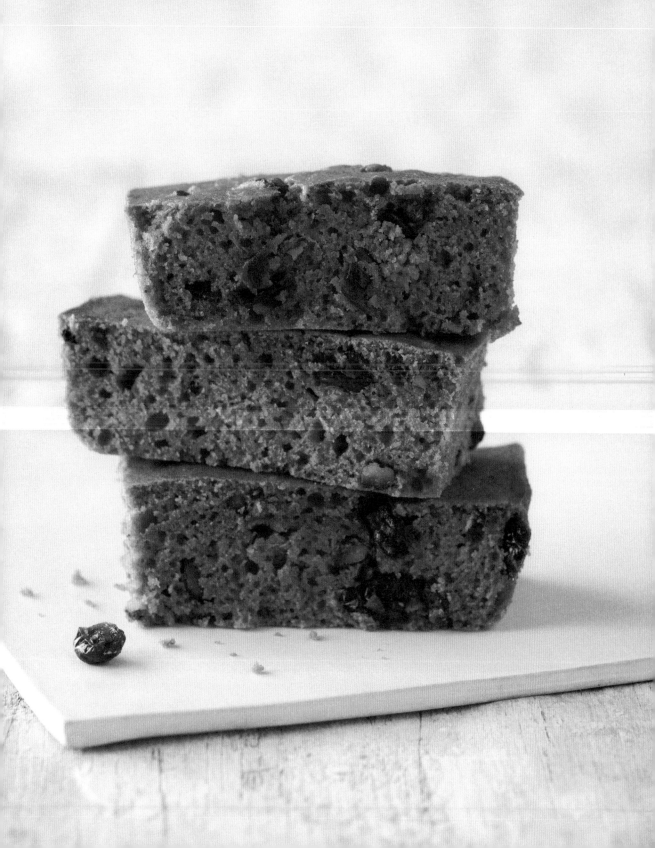

APPLE COBBLER WITH GOLDEN RAISINS AND NUTS

Hazelnut milk and almond flour add sweet, rich, nutty flavor to this fall dessert. Try solo or topped with Whipped Coconut Cream (page 121) or Vanilla Almond Cream (page 119). • **SERVES 4 TO 6**

¾ cup plus 1 tablespoon plain (sweetened) hazelnut milk, divided

2 tablespoons fresh, strained lemon juice, divided

1¾ cups plus 2 tablespoons white whole-wheat flour, divided

½ cup almond flour or meal

¼ cup plus 1 tablespoon Sucanat or brown sugar, divided

1½ teaspoons baking powder

½ teaspoon baking soda

1 teaspoon kosher salt, divided

¾ teaspoon ground cinnamon, divided

6 tablespoons vegan butter (cold), diced

Nonstick cooking spray

5 sweet green or yellow apples, such as Golden Delicious, cored and cut into 1-inch chunks, with peels (about 7 cups)

¼ cup plus 2 tablespoons golden raisins

¼ cup pure maple syrup

2 teaspoons freshly grated lemon zest (about 1 large lemon)

PREHEAT the oven to 375 degrees F. In a medium bowl, whisk the hazelnut milk with 1 tablespoon of the lemon juice, stir, and let sit for 10 minutes.

MEANWHILE, in a large bowl, whisk together 1¾ cups of the white whole-wheat flour, all of the almond flour, ¼ cup of the Sucanat, the baking powder and baking soda, ½ teaspoon of the salt, and ¼ teaspoon of the cinnamon. Whisk well until combined. Add the vegan butter, and, crumble into the dry mix until coarse crumbs form. Pour in all but 1 tablespoon of the hazelnut milk–lemon juice mixture, and form into a ball. Chill.

MEANWHILE, spray a 1½- to 2-quart baking dish (preferably round and relatively shallow) with cooking spray. In a large bowl, mix the apples, raisins, maple syrup, zest, and remaining 2 tablespoons white whole-wheat flour, ½ teaspoon salt, ½ teaspoon cinnamon, and 1 tablespoon lemon juice. Pour into the baking dish.

FORM 6 or 7 large balls of dough, and press over the top of the apple mixture. Brush the tops of the dough rounds with the remaining tablespoon of hazelnut-lemon mixture, and sprinkle with the remaining tablespoon of Sucanat. Place the baking dish onto a rimmed baking sheet, and bake until the fruit is tender, the juices thicken, and the topping is golden brown and cooked through, about 1 hour.

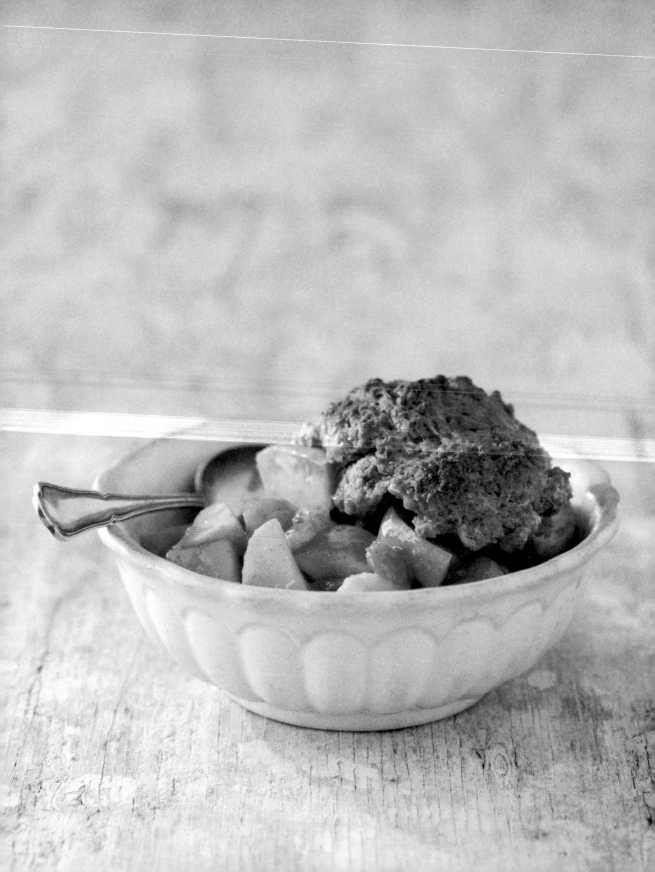

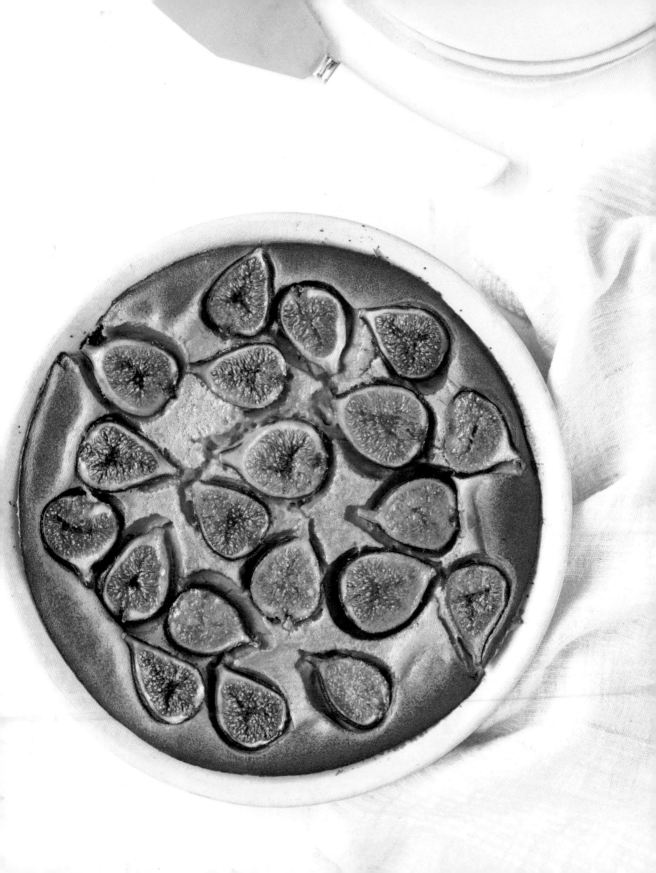

FIG AND HAZELNUT CLAFOUTI WITH ALMOND AND ORANGE

This elegant French dessert is incredibly moist, tender, and pudding-like, despite being whole-grain and free of refined sugar or flour. Try topping it with sweetened hazelnut cream. If using unsweetened hazelnut milk, add one extra tablespoon of Sucanat to the batter.

● **SERVES 6 TO 8**

Nonstick cooking spray

1¼ cups original hazelnut milk (sweetened)

½ cup Sucanat or brown sugar, divided

5 large eggs

2 tablespoons vegetable oil

1 teaspoon pure almond extract

1 teaspoon freshly grated orange zest

⅛ teaspoon kosher salt

½ cup white whole-wheat flour

2 cups halved fresh figs (ideally black
   Mission), stems removed

PREHEAT the oven to 400 degrees F. Grease a 9-inch round baking dish with cooking spray. To a blender, add the hazelnut milk, 6 tablespoons of the Sucanat, eggs, oil, almond extract, orange zest, and salt. Blend until well mixed, about 15 seconds. Add the flour, and blend again until smooth, about 20 seconds (do not overmix). Pour into the greased dish; then sprinkle evenly with the figs and remaining 2 tablespoons Sucanat.

BAKE on the center rack until puffed and golden and a tester poked into the center of the pudding emerges clean, about 45 minutes.

ALTERNATE MILK | CASHEW |

CARDAMOM PUDDING

The Middle East inspired this silky treat, which features cinnamon, cardamom, and orange flower water. • **SERVES 2**

¼ cup plus 2 tablespoons raw unsalted pistachios, soaked for several hours or overnight
1 cup hot water
1 tablespoon plus 2 teaspoons agave nectar

¼ teaspoon ground cinnamon
¼ teaspoon orange flower water or rosewater
⅛ teaspoon kosher salt
⅛ teaspoon ground cardamom
1½ teaspoons cornstarch

RINSE and drain the pistachios. Add to a high-speed blender, along with the fresh hot water and the agave nectar, cinnamon, orange flower water, salt, and cardamom. Puree until smooth, about 1 minute. (Do not strain.)

POUR into a small heavy saucepan. Spoon 2 tablespoons of this mixture into a small bowl, and whisk in the cornstarch until smooth.

BRING the mixture in the saucepan to a boil over medium-high heat. Once the mixture comes to a boil, whisk in the cornstarch mixture, stirring, and boil until the pudding thickens, about 2 minutes. Pour into two 8-ounce dessert glasses or coffee cups. Serve warm or cover, chill until cold (at least 2 hours), and serve cold.

  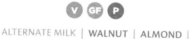

ALTERNATE MILK | **WALNUT** | **ALMOND** |

VANILLA WALNUT PUDDING

For a Mexican version, whisk in a half teaspoon of unsweetened cocoa powder and one sixteenth teaspoon of cayenne pepper. Since walnut milk is lower in fat, boil the mixture for several minutes. Freshly grated lemon zest and ground cinnamon would be nice additions. • **SERVES 1**

¼ cup plus 2 tablespoons raw unsalted
   walnuts, soaked for several hours or
   overnight
1 cup hot water

RINSE and drain the walnuts. Add to a high-speed blender, along with the fresh hot water and the agave nectar, vanilla, and salt. Puree until smooth, about 1 minute. (Do not strain.)

POUR into a small heavy saucepan. Spoon 2 tablespoons of this mixture into a small bowl, and whisk in the cornstarch until smooth.

1 tablespoon plus 2 teaspoons agave nectar
½ teaspoon vanilla extract
⅛ teaspoon kosher salt
1½ teaspoons cornstarch

BRING the mixture in the saucepan to a boil over medium-high heat. Once the mixture comes to a boil, whisk in the cornstarch mixture, stirring, and boil until the pudding thickens, about 8 minutes. Pour into one 8-ounce dessert glass or coffee cup. Serve warm or cover, chill until cold (at least 2 hours), and serve cold.

ALTERNATE MILK | **PECAN** | **HAZELNUT** | **ALMOND** |

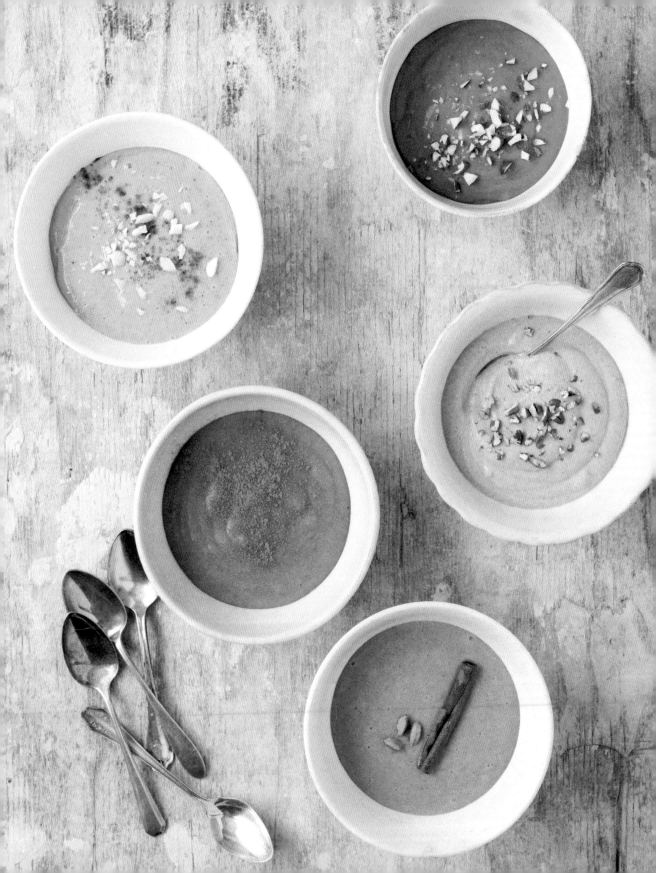

HAZELNUT CINNAMON PUDDING

Note that this pudding is very thick and creamy, even without the cornstarch.
If you're in a rush, just ladle into cups and serve as is, or chill first to serve
the puddings cold. • **SERVES 2**

1 cup blanched unsalted hazelnuts, soaked for
several hours or overnight
1¼ cups hot water
2 tablespoons pure maple syrup

½ teaspoon vanilla extract
¼ teaspoon ground cinnamon
⅛ teaspoon kosher salt
1½ teaspoons cornstarch

RINSE and drain the hazelnuts. Add to a high-speed blender, along with the fresh hot water and the maple syrup, vanilla, cinnamon, and salt. Puree until smooth, about 1 minute. (Do not strain.)

POUR into a small heavy saucepan. Spoon 2 tablespoons of this mixture into a small bowl, and whisk in the cornstarch until smooth.

BRING the mixture in the saucepan to a boil over medium-high heat. Once the mixture comes to a boil, whisk in the cornstarch mixture, stirring, and boil until the pudding thickens slightly more, 1 minute. Pour into two 8-ounce dessert glasses or coffee cups. Serve warm or cover, chill until cold (at least 2 hours), and serve cold.

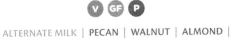

ALTERNATE MILK | PECAN | WALNUT | ALMOND |

CURRIED CASHEW PUDDING

Inspired by the flavors of India, this light golden pudding is rich and exotic. Since the cashew milk is naturally higher in fat, it barely requires the cornstarch. • **SERVES 2**

¼ cup plus 2 tablespoons raw unsalted
   cashews, soaked for several hours or
   overnight
1 cup hot water
1 tablespoon plus 2 teaspoons agave nectar

¼ teaspoon ground cinnamon
¼ teaspoon curry powder
⅛ teaspoon kosher salt
¹⁄₁₆ teaspoon cayenne pepper
1½ teaspoons cornstarch

RINSE and drain the cashews. Add to a high-speed blender, along with the fresh hot water and the agave nectar, cinnamon, curry powder, salt, and cayenne. Puree until smooth, about 1 minute. (Do not strain.)

POUR into a small heavy saucepan. Spoon 2 tablespoons of this mixture into a small bowl, and whisk in the cornstarch until smooth.

BRING the mixture in the saucepan to a boil over medium-high heat. Once the mixture comes to a boil, whisk in the cornstarch mixture, stirring, and boil until the pudding thickens, about 1 minute. Pour into two 8-ounce dessert glasses or coffee cups. Serve warm or cover, chill until cold (at least 2 hours), and serve cold.

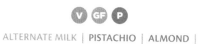

ALTERNATE MILK | **PISTACHIO** | **ALMOND** |

COFFEE ALMOND PUDDING

For a sweet breakfast treat, homemade almond milk mixes with espresso for a morning boost.

● **SERVES 2**

½ cup plus 2 tablespoons raw unsalted almonds, soaked for several hours or overnight

1 cup hot water

2 tablespoons agave nectar

1 teaspoon ground espresso powder

¼ teaspoon almond extract

⅛ teaspoon kosher salt

1½ teaspoons cornstarch

RINSE and drain the almonds. Add to a high-speed blender, along with the fresh hot water and the agave nectar, espresso powder, almond extract, and salt. Puree until smooth, about 1 minute. (Do not strain.)

POUR into a small heavy saucepan. Spoon 2 tablespoons of this mixture into a small bowl, and whisk in the cornstarch until smooth.

BRING the mixture in the saucepan to a boil over medium-high heat. Once the mixture comes to a boil, whisk in the cornstarch mixture, stirring, and boil until the pudding thickens, 2 to 3 minutes. Pour into two 8-ounce dessert glasses or coffee cups. Serve warm or cover, chill until cold (at least 2 hours), and serve cold.

ALTERNATE MILK | HAZELNUT | CASHEW |

KEY LIME "CHEESECAKE" MOUSSE

This sweet-tart mousse tastes like Key lime pie—but dispenses with the traditional sweetened condensed milk. It can be served as pudding, or used to fill the shell of the Vegan Blueberry Cream Tart on page 94. • **MAKES 1½ CUPS (ABOUT 3 SMALL SERVINGS)**

1 cup plain silken tofu, drained (about 8 ounces) and broken up a bit
Flesh of 1 ripe (but not overripe) avocado, about ½ cup
3 tablespoons plus 2 teaspoons agave nectar
2 tablespoons plain unsweetened coconut milk beverage

1 tablespoon fresh, strained Key lime or traditional (Persian) lime juice
1 tablespoon coconut oil
½ teaspoon freshly grated lime zest
½ teaspoon vanilla extract
¼ teaspoon kosher salt

TO a mini food processor, add all of the ingredients. Puree until smooth, about 40 seconds.

LADLE into 3 small cups, and chill.

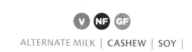

ALTERNATE MILK | CASHEW | SOY |

GRAHAM CRACKER PUDDING

The color of caramel, this low-fat pudding tastes like its namesake! If you don't have graham cracker crumbs, try topping with finely chopped toasted nuts. • **SERVES 4**

2½ cups plain unsweetened flax milk
¼ cup plus 2 tablespoons coconut sugar or brown sugar
2½ tablespoons cornstarch
¼ teaspoon ground cinnamon
¼ teaspoon kosher salt
¼ cup graham cracker crumbs
12 raspberries

ADD the first five ingredients to a small-medium saucepan, and whisk well. Bring to a boil over medium-high heat, whisking occasionally. Boil, whisking frequently, until just thick enough to lightly coat the back of a spoon, 7 to 8 minutes.

LADLE into 4 small coffee cups or parfait glasses, and cover each one with plastic wrap. Chill until further set, at least 2 hours. When ready to serve, divide the graham cracker crumbs and then berries atop each.

Kosher if using kosher graham cracker crumbs

ALTERNATE MILK | CASHEW | SOY |

GREEN TEA–GINGER PUDDING

Look for matcha powder that's bright green and fresh, and be sure to use the yolks only, not the whole eggs. Garnish these puddings with some chopped crystallized ginger. For a variation, infuse the milk with a chopped stalk of fresh lemongrass instead of ginger. • **SERVES 4**

2¼ cups canned full-fat coconut milk (about 1⅓ 13.6-ounce cans), well shaken, divided
½ cup Sucanat or brown sugar
1-inch piece of fresh ginger, sliced
¼ teaspoon kosher salt
3 tablespoons boiling water

1½ tablespoons matcha (ground or powdered Japanese green tea)
3 large egg yolks
1 tablespoon plus 2 teaspoons cornstarch
2 teaspoons vanilla extract

ADD 2 cups of the coconut milk, the Sucanat, ginger, and salt to a small-medium saucepan, and bring to a simmer over medium-high heat (do not let a skin form). Immediately remove from the heat.

MEANWHILE, in a small bowl, whisk together the boiling water and the matcha, and whisk until a velvety mixture forms.

IN a small-medium bowl, whisk together the remaining ¼ cup coconut milk, the yolks, cornstarch, and vanilla. Gradually pour this yolk-cornstarch mixture into the Sucanat-ginger mixture, whisking well. Begin cooking again, bring-

ing to a full boil over medium-high heat, whisking constantly. Immediately reduce the heat to medium low, and simmer, whisking, until thick enough to coat the back of a spoon, about 2 minutes.

SCRAPE the green tea into this thickened milk-egg mixture, and whisk well. Pour through a medium-large fine strainer into a liquid measuring cup or bowl, scraping the pudding out with a rubber spatula. (Wash the spatula and also scrape the bottom of the strainer.) Pour into four 1-cup coffee cups or ramekins, and let cool for 5 minutes. Then directly cover the surface of each pudding with plastic wrap, and chill in the fridge until very cold, at least 2 hours.

MEXICAN CHOCOLATE PUDDING

Hemp milk makes this pudding creamy, and its nutty-grassy flavor stands up to the cocoa and spices. Try topping with candied orange peel. Be sure to use only egg yolks—not the whole eggs—and chile powder that's just ground dried chile pepper, not a blend with salt, cumin, coriander, or other spices. • **SERVES 4**

2¼ cups plain unsweetened hemp milk, divided

½ cup Sucanat or brown sugar

¼ cup plus 1 tablespoon unsweetened cocoa powder

¼ teaspoon kosher salt

⅛ teaspoon ground cinnamon

1/16 teaspoon ancho chile powder

3 large egg yolks

1 tablespoon plus 2 teaspoons cornstarch

2 teaspoons pure vanilla extract

IN a medium saucepan, whisk together 2 cups of the milk, the Sucanat, cocoa, salt, cinnamon, and chile powder. Bring to a simmer over medium-high heat. Immediately remove from the heat.

MEANWHILE, in a small-medium bowl, whisk together the remaining ¼ cup milk, the egg yolks, cornstarch, and vanilla. Slowly whisk this mixture into the spiced cocoa mixture. Place the pot back on the heat. Bring to a full boil over medium-high heat, whisking constantly. Immediately reduce the heat to medium low, and simmer, whisking, until thick, about 3 minutes.

PLACE a handheld fine strainer over a medium bowl and pour the pudding mixture into the strainer, scraping the pudding through with a rubber spatula.

LADLE the pudding mixture into 4 small cups, cover the surface of each directly with plastic wrap, and chill for several hours or overnight.

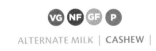

ALTERNATE MILK | CASHEW |

LEMON TAPIOCA PUDDING

Tapioca pudding is the ultimate comfort food: silky and creamy from quick-cooking tapioca balls. This dessert, bright in flavor from the lemon zest and extract, is delicious warm or cold. If you plan on serving it cold, cook for slightly less time, since it will thicken further in the fridge. • **MAKES 2½ CUPS (3 TO 4 SERVINGS)**

3 cups plain unsweetened flax milk
½ cup quick-cooking tapioca
½ cup agave nectar
¼ teaspoon kosher salt

2 large eggs
Zest of 1 lemon (about 1 teaspoon)
½ teaspoon lemon or vanilla extract
About 12 fresh blackberries

ADD the first four ingredients to a medium saucepan, stir well, and bring to a full boil over medium-high heat (watch carefully—don't let a skin form). Immediately reduce the heat to medium low, and simmer, stirring, until slightly thickened, about 5 minutes.

BEAT the eggs in a medium bowl. Very slowly, pour in 1 cup of the hot milk-tapioca mixture, whisking constantly. Pour the egg-milk-tapioca mixture back into the pot with the remaining milk-tapioca mixture. Simmer over medium-low heat, stirring frequently, until the pudding is

thick enough to coat the back of a spoon, about 10 minutes. If you see pieces of cooked egg, strain the pudding through a handheld fine strainer into a medium bowl. Pick out the pieces of egg in the strainer (they will likely be white) and discard. Then, stir the cooked tapioca pearls back into the pudding.

OFF the heat, stir in the zest and extract. Serve warm or chill. If chilling, place plastic wrap directly on the surface, once the pudding has cooled to room temperature. Either way, top with the berries.

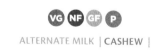

ALTERNATE MILK | CASHEW |

VANILLA ALMOND CREAM

Dollop this velvety cream over desserts, as you would whipped cream or ice cream. If you use nuts with skins, you will see tiny brown flecks, resembling vanilla bean seeds, in the finished cream. For variation, stir in a quarter teaspoon of ground cinnamon. If you'd prefer your cream very sweet, add another tablespoon or two of honey or agave nectar.

● **MAKES A HEAPING 2 CUPS**

1 cup raw unsalted almonds
2 tablespoons agave nectar

½ teaspoon vanilla extract or vanilla bean paste
¼ teaspoon kosher salt

PLACE the nuts in a medium bowl and cover with a couple inches of water. Soak for 8 hours.

RINSE and drain (the nuts will have increased in volume to about 1½ cups), and transfer to a high-speed blender. Add 1 cup fresh water, the honey, vanilla, and salt, and puree until smooth and creamy, about 1 minute.

ALTERNATE CREAM | PISTACHIO | PECAN | WALNUT | | HAZELNUT | MACADAMIA |

BASIC SWEET GLAZE

Drizzle this sweet, decadent glaze over cupcakes or muffins. The whiter the non-dairy milk you use, the whiter the glaze. Don't stir in vanilla extract—it will lend the glaze a light brown tint. • **MAKES ABOUT ½ CUP**

1 cup powdered (confectioner's) sugar

2 tablespoons plain unsweetened coconut milk beverage

COMBINE the powdered sugar and coconut milk beverage in a small bowl and whisk until smooth and glossy.

Nut-free if using coconut milk

ALTERNATE MILK | **CASHEW** | **ALMOND** |

SWEET CREAMY ICING

To transform the above glaze into this slightly thicker, creamier, buttery-tasting icing, just add slightly melted vegan butter. Try it atop cupcakes, muffins, coffee cake, or morning buns. • **MAKES SCANT ⅔ CUP**

1 cup powdered (confectioner's) sugar
2 tablespoons plain unsweetened coconut milk beverage

2 tablespoons vegan butter, barely melted

COMBINE the powdered sugar, coconut milk beverage, and just-melted vegan butter in a small-medium bowl, and whisk well until smooth and glossy.

Nut-free if using coconut milk

ALTERNATE MILK | **CASHEW** | **ALMOND** |

WHIPPED COCONUT CREAM

Use this delicious dessert topping as you would whipped cream or whipped topping.
Feel free to double or triple this recipe. • **MAKES ⅓ CUP**

⅓ cup packed coconut cream, chilled
1 teaspoon sweetener, such as granulated
   sugar

¼ teaspoon vanilla extract or vanilla bean
   paste

COMBINE the chilled coconut cream, sweetener, and vanilla in a standing mixer fitted with a whisk attachment. Beat until creamy, 2 to 3 minutes.

NOTE: Either purchase "coconut cream" (which can be difficult to find), buy cans of full-fat coconut milk free of guar gum (for a higher yield of coconut cream, make sure their contents do not slosh around when shaken), or make your own coconut cream. See page xii for tips on finding coconut cream and guar gum–free canned milk.

If you purchase canned coconut milk or make your own coconut milk, first chill for several hours (also chill the beaters and mixing bowl).

Next, with store-bought canned coconut milk, turn the can upside down, and open with a can opener. Pour off the liquid coconut milk (save for another use), and use the solid coconut cream for this recipe. If you go with homemade coconut milk, spoon off the solid coconut cream that rises to the surface (after chilling for several hours). Save the liquid coconut milk for another use.

Note that it can take two 13.5-ounce cans of coconut milk to yield just ⅓ cup of coconut cream. The yield of coconut cream is similarly low with homemade coconut milk. So, it's always more efficient to begin with packaged coconut cream for whipped coconut cream.

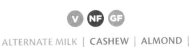

ALTERNATE MILK | CASHEW | ALMOND |

DRINKS

SMOOTHIES

ALMOND

STRAWBERRY-BANANA
BREAKFAST SMOOTHIE

DATE-ALMOND-BANANA
SMOOTHIE

PUMPKIN-MAPLE SMOOTHIE

TROPICAL ORANGE CREAM
SMOOTHIE

AVOCADO-BASIL SMOOTHIE

BANANA–PEANUT BUTTER
SMOOTHIE

COCONUT

BANANA-COCONUT
SMOOTHIE WITH CHOCOLATE
AND ESPRESSO

PIÑA KALE-ADA SMOOTHIE

CHERRY-LIME COCONUT
SMOOTHIE

STRAWBERRY-VANILLA
COCONUT SMOOTHIE

OAT

STRAWBERRY-VANILLA
SMOOTHIE

RICE

QUICK HORCHATA WITH
BANANA

FLAX

SEA SALT–CHOCOLATE
COFFEE FRAPPÉ

HAZELNUT

CHOCOLATE-HAZELNUT
SMOOTHIE

DIETARY CATEGORIES: V VEGAN  VG VEGETARIAN 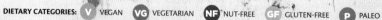 NF NUT-FREE  GF GLUTEN-FREE P PALEO

MILKS

HAZELNUT

HAZELNUT HOT
CHOCOLATE

ALMOND

SPICED CHOCOLATE
MILK

COCONUT

MANGO-SAFFRON MILK

SOY

BLUEBERRY-CARDAMOM
MILK

MATCHA MILK

RICE

RASPBERRY-ROSE MILK

TEAS

ALMOND

LEMON-GINGER MILK
TEA

SWEET ALMOND ROSE
TEA

FLAX

HOT GINGER MILK TEA
WITH TAPIOCA PEARLS

COCONUT

SWEET AND CREAMY
COCONUT CHAI

CASHEW

MATCHA LATTE

STRAWBERRY-BANANA BREAKFAST SMOOTHIE

Thanks to protein powder and flaxseeds, this morning treat is as thick and creamy as a strawberry milkshake. Feel free to halve the recipe. ● **MAKES 4 SCANT CUPS (4 SERVINGS)**

2 cups plain unsweetened almond milk

1½ cups frozen strawberries (unsweetened)

1 large very ripe banana

8 pitted dates

1 tablespoon unflavored protein powder (such as rice or soy)

1 tablespoon flaxseeds (whole or ground)

1 teaspoon vanilla extract

⅛ teaspoon kosher salt

ADD all of the ingredients to a high-speed blender and puree until smooth, about 40 seconds.

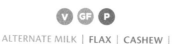

ALTERNATE MILK | **FLAX** | **CASHEW** |

ALMOND

DATE-ALMOND-BANANA SMOOTHIE

This one-step vegan smoothie is sweet, orangey, and delicious. • **MAKES 1½ CUPS (1 SERVING)**

1 cup plain unsweetened almond milk

1 very ripe medium banana

4 pitted dates

2 ice cubes

2 tablespoons strained fresh orange juice

½ teaspoon pure almond or vanilla extract

⅛ teaspoon ground cardamom or cinnamon

⅛ teaspoon kosher salt

ADD all of the ingredients to a high-speed blender and blend until smooth, about 30 seconds.

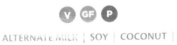

ALTERNATE MILK | SOY | COCONUT |

PUMPKIN-MAPLE SMOOTHIE

Creamy and sweet, this smoothie tastes like pumpkin pie. If you don't love nutmeg or ginger,
reduce those quantities to one-sixteenth teaspoon. ● **MAKES ABOUT 4 CUPS (4 SERVINGS)**

2 cups plain unsweetened almond milk

1 cup canned unsweetened pumpkin puree

1 large very ripe banana

3 tablespoons pure maple syrup

1 tablespoon ground flaxseeds

1 tablespoon creamy almond butter

¼ teaspoon kosher salt

¼ teaspoon ground cinnamon

⅛ teaspoon ground nutmeg

⅛ teaspoon ground cloves

⅛ teaspoon ground ginger

ADD all of the ingredients to a high-speed blender and blend until smooth, about 1 minute.

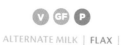

ALTERNATE MILK | **FLAX** |

TROPICAL ORANGE CREAM SMOOTHIE

Imagine orange cream pops, with their vanilla ice cream center and orange sorbet exterior. These smoothies are a healthier, dairy-free version—with protein powder added to make them more substantial. ● **MAKES 3½ CUPS (ABOUT 3 SERVINGS)**

1½ cups cubed frozen pineapple

1½ cups cubed frozen mango

1 cup plain unsweetened almond milk

½ cup strained fresh orange juice

3 tablespoons unflavored protein powder (such as rice or pea)

3 tablespoons agave nectar

1 teaspoon vanilla extract

⅛ teaspoon kosher salt

BLEND all of the ingredients in a high-speed blender until relatively smooth, about 40 seconds.

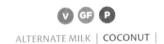

ALTERNATE MILK | **COCONUT** |

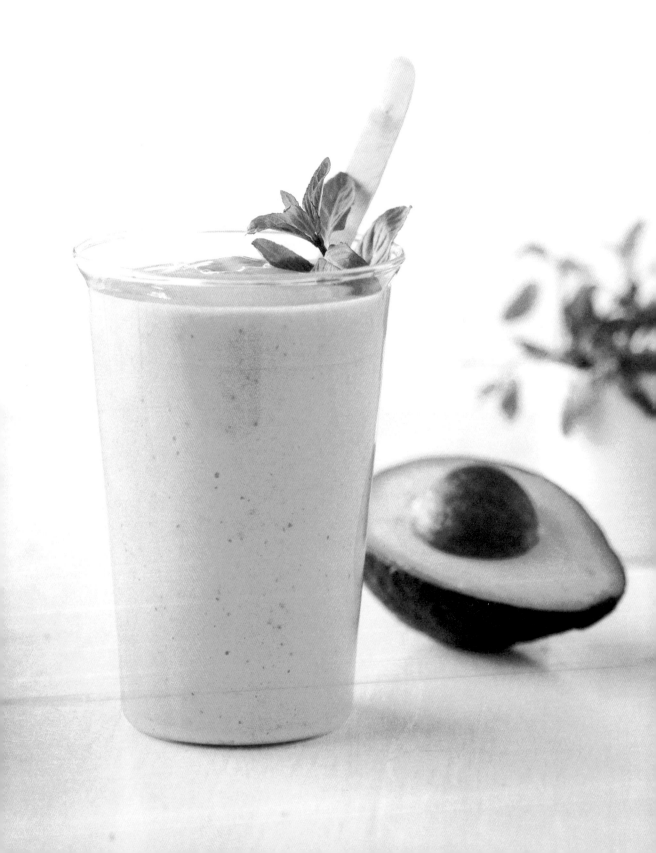

AVOCADO-BASIL SMOOTHIE

Thick and rich, this vegan smoothie is like a gorgeous green milkshake! Select an avocado that gives only a tiny bit when squeezed. Opt for frozen pineapple—it yields a creamy, icy consistency. ● **MAKES 1½ CUPS (1 TO 2 SERVINGS)**

1 cup plain unsweetened almond milk

Flesh of 1 slightly ripe avocado

⅓ cup cubed frozen pineapple

3 tablespoons strained fresh orange juice

2 tablespoons agave nectar

8 fresh basil (or fresh mint) leaves

⅛ teaspoon kosher salt

ADD all of the ingredients to a high-speed blender, and blend until smooth, about 30 seconds.

ALTERNATE MILK | RICE | COCONUT

BANANA–PEANUT BUTTER SMOOTHIE

Try blending in the morning, and drinking later on—this smoothie will hold. If your bananas are extremely ripe and sweet, you can probably get by with only three tablespoons of agave nectar. ● **MAKES 6 CUPS (6 SERVINGS)**

3 cups plain unsweetened almond milk

3 large very ripe bananas

½ cup plus 2 tablespoons (salted) creamy or chunky peanut butter

¼ cup agave nectar, or to taste

4 ice cubes

1 tablespoon flaxseeds (whole or ground)

2 teaspoons vanilla extract

ADD all of the ingredients to a high-speed blender and puree until smooth, about 40 seconds.

ALTERNATE MILK | SOY |

BANANA-COCONUT SMOOTHIE WITH CHOCOLATE AND ESPRESSO

This smoothie melds coffee, coconut, chocolate, and banana.

● **MAKES ABOUT 5 CUPS (4 TO 5 SERVINGS)**

3 cups plain unsweetened coconut milk beverage (not canned)

2½ cups mashed very ripe bananas (about 3 large)

2 tablespoons coconut oil

1 tablespoon plus 1 teaspoon unsweetened cocoa powder

1 tablespoon plus 1 teaspoon agave nectar

1 tablespoon espresso powder

1 tablespoon shredded unsweetened coconut

4 ice cubes

1 teaspoon vanilla extract

½ teaspoon kosher salt

ADD all of the ingredients to a high-speed blender and blend until smooth, about 1 minute. Serve immediately.

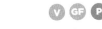

ALTERNATE MILK | CASHEW | HEMP |

PIÑA KALE-ADA SMOOTHIE

This smoothie captures the flavors of a piña colada—without alcohol, or sugar, or fat-laden cream of coconut. Plus, you'll derive the health benefits of kale and protein powder.

● **MAKES ABOUT 5 CUPS (5 SERVINGS)**

2 cups plain unsweetened coconut milk

2 cups cubed frozen pineapple

1 cup thinly sliced fresh kale leaves
   (ribs removed)

2 tablespoons unflavored protein powder
   (such as soy or rice)

1 tablespoon agave nectar

1 tablespoon fresh, strained lime juice

⅛ teaspoon kosher salt

PUREE all of the ingredients in a high-speed blender until smooth, about 40 seconds.

ALTERNATE MILK | **ALMOND** | **SOY** |

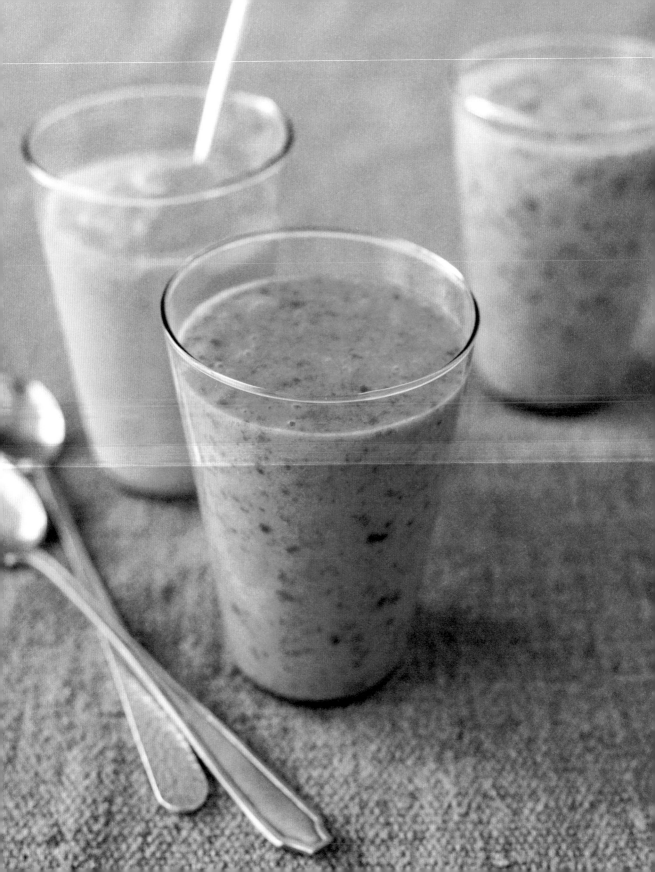

CHERRY-LIME COCONUT SMOOTHIE

In this colorful smoothie, fresh lime juice adds a hint of tartness to balance out the sweet cherries. Coconut milk supplies richness and creaminess.

● **MAKES 4 CUPS**

1 pound frozen sweet cherries
13.5-ounce can coconut milk (full-fat)

2 tablespoons agave nectar or honey
Scant 2 tablespoons fresh lime juice, strained

ADD all of the ingredients to a blender, and puree until smooth, about 1 minute. Serve immediately.

ALTERNATE MILK | ALMOND | CASHEW |

STRAWBERRY-VANILLA COCONUT SMOOTHIE

Seek out small, local berries for this smoothie.

● **MAKES ABOUT 5 CUPS**

4 cups hulled fresh strawberries, preferably
  local

2 cups plain unsweetened coconut milk
  beverage

3 large ice cubes

3 tablespoons agave nectar

1 teaspoon vanilla extract

⅛ teaspoon salt

ADD all of the ingredients to a high-speed blender, and puree until smooth, about 1 minute.

STRAWBERRY-VANILLA SMOOTHIE

This high-fiber, protein-rich smoothie tastes like strawberry ice cream.

● **MAKES 3½ CUPS (ABOUT 3 SERVINGS)**

2¼ cups plain unsweetened oat milk

1 cup frozen unsweetened strawberries

1 cup raw old-fashioned or quick oats

6 pitted dates (or a few tablespoons agave nectar)

3 tablespoons unflavored protein powder (such as rice or pea)

1 teaspoon vanilla extract

⅛ teaspoon kosher salt

BLEND all of the ingredients in a high-speed blender until relatively smooth, about 40 seconds.

Gluten-free if using gluten-free oats

ALTERNATE MILK | RICE |

QUICK HORCHATA WITH BANANA

Horchata is a Mexican drink consisting of raw long-grain white rice, water, milk, cinnamon, and vanilla. Traditionally a time-intensive recipe that calls for soaking the ingredients for a few hours, this shortcut version takes mere minutes, thanks to rice milk. Bananas add creaminess. • **MAKES 3½ CUPS (ABOUT 3 SERVINGS)**

2 cups plain unsweetened rice milk

2 large ripe bananas

2 tablespoons unflavored protein powder
   (such as pea or rice)

2 tablespoons agave nectar

2 teaspoons vanilla extract

½ teaspoon ground cinnamon

3 ice cubes

ADD all of the ingredients to a high-speed blender and blend until smooth, about 30 seconds. Serve immediately over ice.

ALTERNATE MILK | ALMOND | COCONUT |

SEA SALT–CHOCOLATE COFFEE FRAPPÉ

For a coffeehouse presentation, dollop with coconut cream. Use a vegetable peeler and chocolate bar to form chocolate shavings. • **MAKES 3½ CUPS (ABOUT 2 LARGE SERVINGS)**

2 tablespoons ground coffee

2 cups ice cubes

1 cup plain unsweetened flax milk

¼ cup agave nectar

¼ cup unsweetened cocoa powder

1 teaspoon vanilla extract

¼ teaspoon sea salt

Optional for garnish: coconut cream and semisweet or dark chocolate shavings

BREW coffee using 1 (8-ounce) cup water and all of the ground coffee. Chill.

COMBINE ¾ cup of the coffee with the remaining ingredients in a high-speed blender, and puree until smooth (with small pieces of ice), about 30 seconds. Serve immediately.

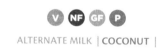

ALTERNATE MILK | COCONUT |

CHOCOLATE-HAZELNUT SMOOTHIE

Chocolate plus hazelnuts. Need I say more? Banana and protein powder make this decadent-tasting smoothie creamy and nourishing. • **MAKES 3½ CUPS (ABOUT 3 SERVINGS)**

2 cups plain hazelnut milk (sweetened)

2 very ripe large bananas

¼ cup unsweetened cocoa powder

¼ cup unflavored protein powder
  (such as pea or rice)

4 ice cubes

2 tablespoons agave nectar

1 teaspoon hazelnut or vanilla extract

⅛ teaspoon kosher salt

ADD all of the ingredients to a high-speed blender and puree until smooth, about 30 seconds.

  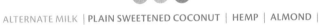

ALTERNATE MILK | PLAIN SWEETENED COCONUT | HEMP | ALMOND |

HAZELNUT HOT CHOCOLATE

Look for hazelnut extract—it adds a rich, deep, nutty flavor.
Try dolloping with coconut cream. • **MAKES 4 CUPS (3 TO 4 SERVINGS)**

1 quart plain hazelnut milk (sweetened)
⅓ cup unsweetened cocoa powder
2 ounces semisweet chocolate, chopped
2 tablespoons agave nectar

2 teaspoons hazelnut or vanilla extract
1 teaspoon vanilla extract (3 teaspoons total,
** if vanilla extract is used above)**
⅛ teaspoon kosher salt

ADD the hazelnut milk to a medium saucepan, and bring to a boil over medium-high heat. Turn off the heat and whisk in the remaining ingredients, scraping the bottom of the pot with a wooden spoon to incorporate all of the melted chocolate. Ladle into mugs and serve immediately. (If reheating later, stir well before serving.)

ALTERNATE MILK | COCONUT | HEMP |

SPICED CHOCOLATE MILK

This super chocolaty milk is way more flavorful than the version you remember from childhood. To appeal to young kids, omit the spices. • **MAKES ABOUT 1 CUP (1 SERVING)**

1 cup plus 2 tablespoons plain unsweetened almond milk

1 ounce semisweet chocolate, broken up

1 tablespoon unsweetened cocoa powder

1 tablespoon agave nectar

1 cinnamon stick

3 whole cloves

2 cardamom pods

ADD all of the ingredients to a small sauce-pan, whisk well, and bring to a simmer over medium-high heat. Simmer until the cocoa powder and chocolate dissolve, whisking, about 3 minutes.

STRAIN into a small-medium bowl, cover, and chill until cold, about 1 hour. Remove the spices, pour into a glass, and serve cold.

Vegan if using vegan chocolate; nut-free if using nut-free milk

ALTERNATE MILK | CASHEW | HEMP |

MANGO-SAFFRON MILK

Indian mango lassis (yogurt smoothies) inspired this yellow-orange infused milk. If you don't like cardamom, omit it or substitute ground cinnamon. In addition to employing the syrup in these beverages, try it spooned over non-dairy rice pudding or yogurt.

● **MAKES ½ CUP SYRUP AND 2 CUPS FLAVORED MILK (2 SERVINGS)**

1 cup frozen or fresh mango chunks
2 tablespoons plus 2 teaspoons agave nectar
¼ teaspoon saffron threads

1½ cups plain unsweetened non-dairy milk,
  especially coconut or rice, chilled

ADD the mango, agave nectar, and saffron, plus 2 tablespoons water, to a small saucepan, and bring to a simmer over medium-high heat. Reduce the heat to low, and simmer until the mango is very soft, about 3 minutes.

SCRAPE the contents of the pan into a mini food processor, and puree until very smooth, about 1 minute. Place a fine strainer over a liquid

measuring cup, and strain well, stirring the inside contents of the strainer to get all the liquid out. Then, clean the spoon, and scrape the bottom of the strainer until you glean all of the syrup (you should end up with ½ cup).

FOR each serving of milk, combine ¼ cup syrup with ¾ cup of milk, and whisk well. Serve cold.

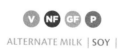

ALTERNATE MILK | SOY |

BLUEBERRY-CARDAMOM MILK

To prepare this infused blue-purple milk, first make syrup (which can also be used as a dessert sauce). If you don't like cardamom, omit it or substitute with ground cinnamon.

● **MAKES ¾ CUP SYRUP AND 3 CUPS FLAVORED MILK (3 SERVINGS)**

1 cup frozen or fresh blueberries
2 tablespoons agave nectar
⅛ teaspoon ground cardamom

2¼ cups any plain unsweetened non-dairy milk, especially soy or rice, chilled

ADD the berries, agave nectar, and cardamom plus 2 tablespoons water to a small saucepan, and bring to a simmer over medium-high heat. Reduce the heat to low, and simmer until the berries are very soft, about 2 minutes.

SCRAPE the contents of the pan into a mini food processor, and puree until very smooth, about 1 minute. Place a fine strainer over a

liquid measuring cup, and strain well, stirring the contents inside of the strainer well to get all the liquid out. Then, clean the spoon and scrape the bottom of the strainer until you glean all of the syrup (you should end up with ¾ cup).

FOR each serving of milk, combine ¼ cup syrup with ¾ cup of the milk, and whisk well. Serve.

ALTERNATE MILK | PISTACHIO | COCONUT |

MATCHA MILK

Matcha is finely ground high-quality Japanese green tea with grassy and floral flavor notes.
Whisking it with boiling water first helps it dissolve. • **MAKES ABOUT 1 CUP (1 SERVING)**

¼ cup boiling water

1 teaspoon bright-green matcha powder

¾ cup plain unsweetened non-dairy milk,
  especially soy milk, chilled

1 tablespoon agave nectar

¼ teaspoon vanilla extract

IN a liquid measuring cup, whisk together the boiling water and the matcha, and pour into a small fine strainer set over a medium mug (stir the inside contents of the strainer and scrape the underside to glean all of the liquid). Add the remaining ingredients, whisk well, and chill. Serve cold.

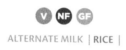

ALTERNATE MILK | RICE |

RASPBERRY-ROSE MILK

Strawberry milk inspired this much more sophisticated magenta-hued beverage.
After preparing one recipe of the milk, you will have two tablespoons of syrup left,
just enough as a dessert topping for one.

● **MAKES ¼ CUP PLUS 2 TABLESPOONS SYRUP AND 1 TO 1¼ CUPS MILK (1 SERVING)**

1 cup frozen or fresh raspberries

3 tablespoons agave nectar

1 tablespoon dried organic rosebuds

¾ cup plain unsweetened non-dairy milk,
especially rice or almond, chilled

ADD the berries, agave nectar, and rosebuds, plus 2 tablespoons water, to a small saucepan, and bring to a simmer over medium-high heat. Reduce the heat to low, and simmer until the berries are very soft, about 4 minutes.

WITH a potato masher, mash until almost smooth. Scrape the contents of the pan into a fine strainer set over a liquid measuring cup.

Strain well, stirring the inside contents of the strainer to get all the liquid out. Then, clean the spoon and scrape the bottom of the strainer until you glean all of the syrup (you should end up with ¼ cup plus 2 tablespoons).

FOR each serving of milk, combine ¼ cup of syrup with ¾ cup of milk (or 1 cup, for a more subtle version), and whisk well. Serve cold.

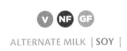

ALTERNATE MILK | SOY |

LEMON-GINGER MILK TEA

I love to prepare this citrusy tea for my sons when they're sick.
For a less sweet drink, reduce the syrup. • **MAKES ABOUT 1¾ CUPS (2 TO 3 SERVINGS)**

2 cups plain unsweetened almond milk
¼ cup pure maple syrup or agave nectar
1-inch piece of fresh ginger, thinly sliced

Zest of 1 lemon (yellow part only, no white pith)
1 green tea sachet or bag (caffeinated or decaffeinated)

ADD all of the ingredients to a medium saucepan, and bring to a simmer over high heat. Turn off the heat and let sit for 5 minutes. Strain into a 2-cup or larger liquid measuring cup with a spout. Pour into cups, and serve.

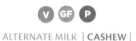

ALTERNATE MILK | CASHEW |

SWEET ALMOND ROSE TEA

A real ambrosia, this tea is ideal with cookies or before bedtime.

● **MAKES ABOUT 2 CUPS (2 SERVINGS)**

2 cups plain unsweetened almond milk
¼ cup dried organic rose petals

2 tablespoons agave nectar (or honey)

ADD the ingredients to a small saucepan, and bring to a boil over medium-high heat. Immediately cover and simmer over low. Simmer for 5 minutes, strain into a bowl, and ladle into 2 mugs.

ALTERNATE MILK | RICE |

HOT GINGER MILK TEA WITH TAPIOCA PEARLS

I'm obsessed with bubble tea—for good reason. The bubbles are actually cooked tapioca pearls, which resemble black marbles and are soft and slightly spongy in texture (in a good way!). Customize this recipe by using decaffeinated or green tea. Feel free to vary the type of tapioca pearls you use. If you pick a different type, follow the package directions for cooking them. ● **MAKES 2½ CUPS (2 SERVINGS)**

½ cup uncooked (quick-cooking) black tapioca pearls
2 cups plain unsweetened flax milk
1-inch piece of fresh ginger, chopped

2 unflavored black tea bags or sachets, such as English Breakfast or Darjeeling
¼ cup agave nectar (or to taste)

FILL a medium saucepan two-thirds full of water, cover, and bring to a boil over high heat. Stir in the tapioca pearls, and boil for 5 minutes. Reduce the heat to medium, and simmer until tender, about 5 minutes. Drain in a colander in the sink.

MEANWHILE, add the flax milk and ginger to a small-medium saucepan, and bring to a boil over

medium-high heat. Immediately add the tea bags, reduce the heat to low, and simmer for 5 minutes. Strain into a liquid measuring cup with a spout (discard the tea bags and ginger). Stir in the cooked tapioca pearls and agave nectar. Add to 2 teacups, serving with spoons.

 GF P

Vegan if vegan tapioca pearls are used

ALTERNATE MILK | SOY | COCONUT |

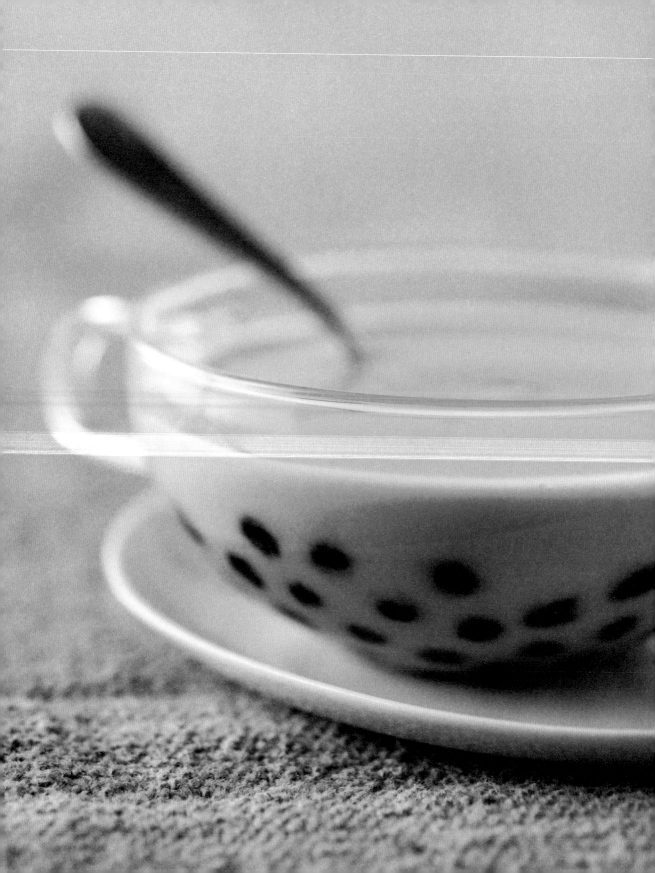

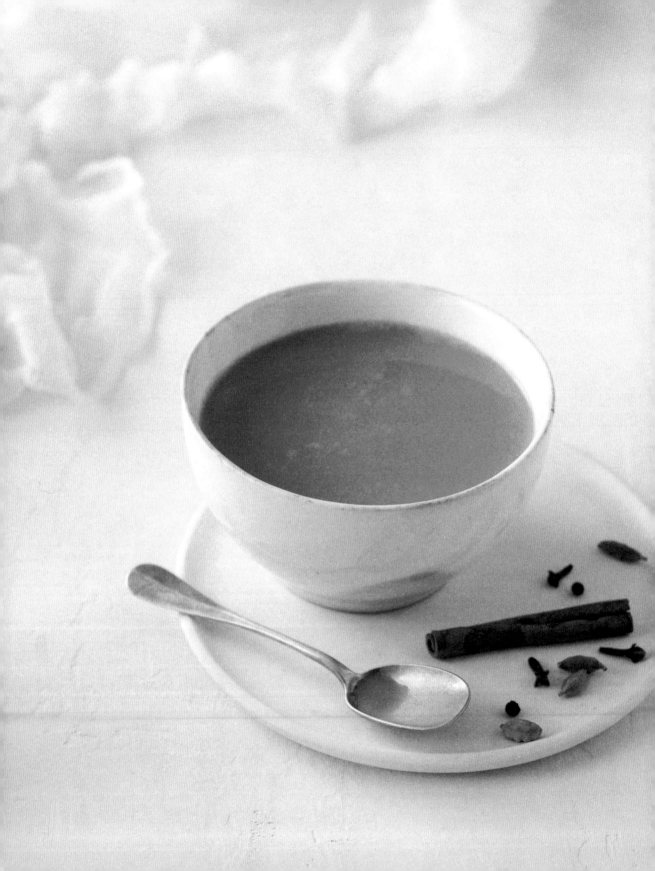

SWEET AND CREAMY COCONUT CHAI

Cocoa nibs and coconut milk lend complexity to this warm spiced Indian tea. For a caffeine-free version, use decaffeinated black tea bags. • **MAKES ABOUT FIVE 8-OUNCE CUPS (5 SERVINGS)**

4 cups plain unsweetened almond milk
1-inch piece of fresh ginger, thinly sliced
16 whole cardamom pods, crushed
10 whole cloves
1 cinnamon stick
6 whole peppercorns (black, green,
   or pink)

½ teaspoon ground cacao nibs or
   unsweetened cocoa
6 unflavored black tea bags or sachets, such as
   English Breakfast or Darjeeling
1 cup canned light coconut milk (about
   ½ can), well shaken (at room temperature)
¼ cup plus 2 tablespoons agave nectar

ADD the almond milk to a medium-large saucepan, and bring to a simmer over medium-high heat.

MEANWHILE, place the ginger, cardamom, cloves, cinnamon, peppercorns, and cacao onto a medium piece of cheesecloth. Form into a bundle, and tie with kitchen twine.

ONCE the almond milk has come to a steady simmer, stir in the spice bundle and tea bags. Cover the pot and turn the heat to low. Simmer for 5 minutes. Remove and discard the spice bundle and tea bags. Turn off the heat and let the pot sit on the hot burner for 5 minutes. Stir in the milk and agave. Ladle the warm chai into mugs, and serve.

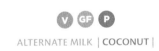

ALTERNATE MILK | COCONUT |

MATCHA LATTE

Matcha is ground high-grade Japanese green tea with a floral and grassy flavor. This latte is velvety, sweet, and a gorgeous springy green hue. I highly recommend the Aerolatte milk frother, which costs about twenty dollars, for homemade lattes. • **MAKES 1 SERVING**

**1½ teaspoons strained matcha
(1 teaspoon for a milder cup)**
2 tablespoons very hot water

1 cup plain unsweetened cashew milk
1 tablespoon plus ½ teaspoon agave nectar
¼ teaspoon vanilla extract

WHISK together the matcha with the very hot water until mostly smooth (a few tiny lumps will remain). Meanwhile, heat the cashew milk in a 12-ounce mug in the microwave or in a small saucepan on the stovetop until very hot.

SCRAPE the matcha mixture into the hot cashew milk. Add the agave nectar and vanilla. Froth with an Aerolatte or other handheld battery-powered milk frother until very frothy. Serve immediately.

ALTERNATE MILK | COCONUT | SOY | ALMOND |

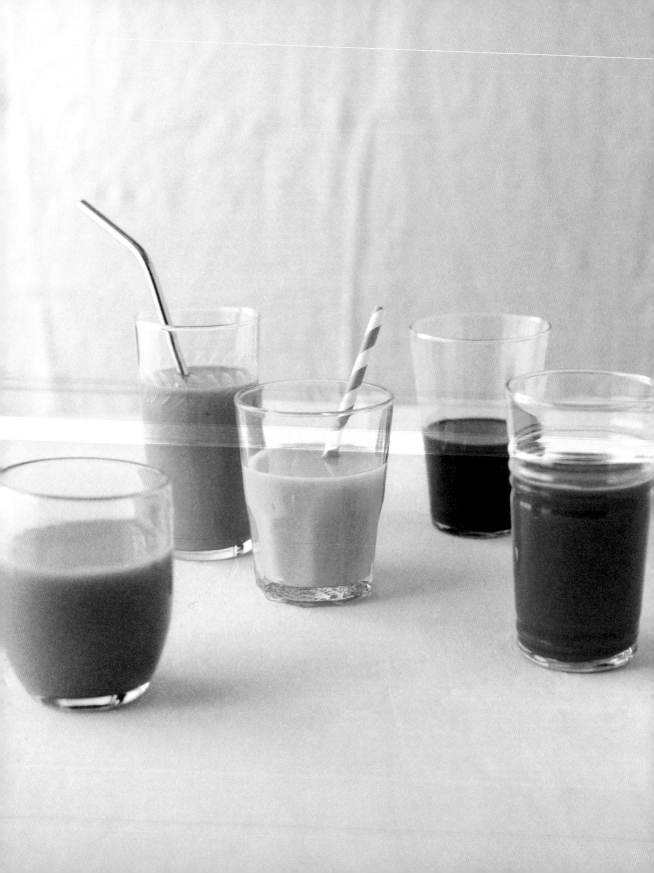

ACKNOWLEDGMENTS

Thanks to my friends and colleagues Jackie Mills, MS, RD; Alia Hanna Habib; and Jenna Helwig for encouraging me to pursue this idea and find a home for it. Thanks to my agent, Jenni Ferrari-Adler, who found that home, and to Donna Loffredo, Sara DeLozier, Leslie Meredith, and everyone at Atria for their enthusiasm and trust in my vision. My gratitude extends to the entire team responsible for the gorgeous book you have in your hands, among them photographer Sabra Krock and food stylist Molly Shuster. I'm grateful to David Katz, MD; Guy Crosby; Kayleen St. John, MS, RD; and friend and colleague Nicole Jones, who helped me understand the nutritional aspects of non-dairy milks (not a simple subject). Thanks to Breville for sending me two unbelievable appliances with which to play: "The Boss™" High-Velocity Blender and The Sous Chef food processor. Much gratitude to my mother, Harriet, for conducting extensive research. Finally, thanks to my amazing husband, Koby, for all of his editing, love, and support.

DAIRY-FREE RESOURCES

General resources

www.thenewmilks.com

www.godairyfree.org

www.glutenfreeandmore.com

www.foodallergy.org

www.milkfreepantry.com

www.ohsheglows.com

Nutrition and Food Science

www.naturalgourmetinstitute.com

www.davidkatzmd.com

www.cookingscienceguy.com

Dairy-free milk and yogurt

www.sodeliciousdairyfree.com

www.silk.com

www.bluediamond.com

www.califiafarms.com

www.livingharvest.com

www.pearlsoymilk.com

www.organicvalley.coop

www.tastethedream.com

www.edenfoods.com

www.facebook.com/Suzies.Natural.Products

www.pacificfoods.com

www.facebook.com/nativeforest

www.facebook.com/Idorganic

www.thaikitchen.com

Dairy-free butter

www.earthbalancenatural.com

Dairy-free cheese and cream cheese

www.daiyafoods.com

www.goveggiefoods.com

www.cheezehound.com

www.treelinecheese.com

www.miyokoskitchen.com

www.dr-cow.com

www.tofutti.com

www.followyourheart.com

www.riverdelcheese.com (dairy-free cheese shop in Brooklyn, NY)

vtopiancheeses.com (dairy-free cheese shop in Portland, OR)

www.vromage.com (dairy-free cheese shop in West Hollywood, CA)

Dairy-free ice cream

www.stevesicecream.com (some flavors)

www.gourmetsorbet.com

www.coconutbliss.com

www.tastethedream.com

www.vanleeuwenicecream.com (some flavors)

www.dfmavens.com

www.tofutti.com

www.fomuicecream.com (vegan ice cream shop in Boston, MA)

www.sweetritual.com (dairy-free ice cream shop in Austin, TX)

INDEX

ABOUT THE AUTHOR

DINA CHENEY is also the author of *Mug Meals, Meatless All Day, Year-Round Slow Cooker, Williams-Sonoma New Flavors for Salads*, and *Tasting Club*. She writes and develops recipes for numerous publications and styles and photographs much of her work. A graduate of Columbia University and The Institute of Culinary Education, Dina is on Instagram (@thenewmilks) and www.dinacheney.com. Visit her dairy-free resource site: www.thenewmilks.com.